Practice Matters

THE EARLY YEARS OF MODERN
GENERAL PRACTICE WITHIN THE NHS

ANDREW WILLIS

Saighton Books

CHESTER, UK

Saighton Books
Chester, UK
www.practice-matters.co.uk

Book Layout © 2014 BookDesignTemplates.com

Practice Matters/**Andrew Willis**. 1st edn
ISBN 978-0-9956555-1-5

To Eunice, our family, and my parents John and Jean

When an old man dies, a library burns to the ground

– AFRICAN PROVERB

CONTENTS

PREFACE

Practice Matters is the memoir of a family doctor whose National Health Service (NHS) career lasted from 1970 to 2006. These were years of unprecedented change in medical opportunity, buildings, personnel, available technologies and the professional structure of general practice. There has never been such a dynamic period in the history of UK medical practice.

It is a personal story, but at the same time it describes the broader context: the evolution of UK general practice from the apothecaries' dispensaries to the complex medical centres of the 21st century.

So why a book? Why not a website or blog? Although innovations in information technology occur at an ever-increasing pace, it is likely that future historians and the curious will still turn, at least in part, to the printed narrative for accounts of the development of general practice, the lives of those working within it, and of the NHS as an organisation. There is documented research aplenty about the mechanics of medical practice, but far fewer personal accounts of what it has been like to work in the NHS at any particular time. I hope this book serves as a contribution to that literature.

As a memoir, *Practice Matters* contains personal opinion and inevitable bias. That said, a genuine attempt has been made to provide balance concerning contentious issues. I apologise in advance for any errors or omissions of fact, and particularly for any offence caused by what I have written. That was not my intention.

Inevitably, associated material could not be included in the book, either through lack of space or because a printed document is no longer available. I will be including it within an archive on www.practice-matters.co.uk.

ACKNOWLEDGEMENTS

I have been drafting this book for 10 years. Many, many people have contributed to its contents, but a few stand out. I would like to thank them for the help they gave me during my career.

My partners over the years: Jim Mitchell, Chris Elliott-Binns, Michael Woolmore, Allan Leroy, Judith Reader, John Rickerby, Simon Gregory, Claire Jenks, Mahmood Kausar, and Ann Wood. Wonderful family doctors, which is my highest compliment. It was a very real privilege to work with you.

Bill McQuillan, Mike Sobanja, and Keith Oswin at and beyond Northampton Health Authority. Together we did some amazing things in difficult times.

My sons, Mark and Paul, and my daughter-in-law Caroline, all of whom as students undertook invaluable research and development projects for the practice. Earlier, as children, the boys were the only people light enough to walk on the glass roof at Billing Road each summer, spraying it with white sunshade. Staff and patients alike were grateful for that.

Alan Birchall, Quentin Shaw, Ron Singer, and all the committee of the National Association of Commissioning GPs. I always said that accounts of the history of the NHS should acknowledge these remarkable pioneers, and to work with them was one of the greatest highlights of my career.

Les Zendle at Kaiser Permanente, Southern California, who arranged and hosted my visit there for a week in 2002, an experience that proved to be a major influence on my subsequent thinking.

Our wonderful practice staff, with a special mention for the managers Joyce Hall, Julie Trew, Maggie Hoppitt, and Justin Pearce, and the IT manager Carol Hyde.

Chris Ham, Peter Spurgeon, and Penny Mullen – at the time all at Health Services Management Centre, University of Birmingham. My advisers and research supervisors, they showed me what academia is all about.

The thousands of patients at the practice for providing such inspiration and huge job satisfaction.

The many other practices in the country that pushed the boundaries of the possible and collectively produced modern general practice, the linchpin of a successful future NHS. Our practice was merely an example of the whole.

Others have helped turn the text into reality. Rosie Rushton for a decade of patient help and encouragement, and my brother James for persuading me to stop rewriting it over and over again, and actually publish it. My family are grateful to you for that! And of course, my professional team – the ever-patient editor Sonia Cutler, Emma Hardy who designed the cover, and Nicola King, who produced the index. I shudder to think what the book would have been like without you three. No doubt you do too!

If anyone can identify the artist of the painting on page 23, I would be delighted to hear from them, so that I can fully acknowledge her in the future. My thanks also to the National Archives (www.nationalarchives.gov.uk) for providing the excerpt from the Dawson Report shown on page 64. Unless otherwise stated, the photographs used in the book were taken by me.

My wife Eunice was one of the first computer widows in the early 1980s yet a rock of encouragement as I explored the extraneous rivulets of my career. She was widowed again when we retired, this time by an erstwhile author, his research, and endless drafts. Thank you for your unstinting support over the 10 years I have been writing this book. Perhaps, now, at last …

And finally, Tom King, FRCS, without whom, as they say, none of this would have been possible. I shall forever be in your debt.

INTRODUCTION

Until the 1970s and 1980s, general practice was the poor relation of the NHS. It had been seen by many as subordinate to hospitals, a minor illness service staffed by an uncontrolled group of clinicians of little value other than to act as referral gatekeepers for the expensive hospitals.

But then things changed, and to a remarkable extent. Four decades later, the most dynamic and successful part of the NHS is not its hospitals, but its general practices. The actions of recent governments – of any political persuasion – demonstrate that even politicians realise that general practice is now the pivot, the playmaker of the health service.

So, what was it that changed?

The reason the NHS is so popular is that it is rooted on a set of unarguably appropriate, sound principles: fairness, the inclusion of the whole population without financial restriction at the point of access, and equity, that is, treatment according to relative need.

That equity of provision is what distinguishes the NHS from crude markets, with their inherent losers and winners. Population-wide healthcare is not a simple commodity; in the case of the NHS, those who argue otherwise inevitably deny its founding principles.

Unlike cruder systems, it is based on the provision of services to populations. Most obviously, there is the whole country, but there are smaller, constituent populations such as local communities, those attending a hospital, and most importantly those registered with a general practice. It is the cohesion of these subpopulations, their recognition of each other, and their interoperability that defines an effective national health service.

General practice interleaves care of the individual with that of its registered list. That list is nothing less than the building block on which the NHS has been built. Yet, it is only since the 1970s and 1980s that practices have been able to turn into reality the full, latent potential of the NHS. A practice is responsible for providing this defined population with the three elements of medical care: short-term care, preventive measures, and the management of continuing, chronic conditions, and to do so inclusively and according to relative need. No other component of the health service has such a broad brief. In short, a general practice is the NHS in microcosm.

This book explores and explains the changes that have turned the potential into reality. It paints a broader picture of the NHS than television's flashing lights, ambulances, and operating theatres with their earnest staff in blue pyjamas. Such aspects represent a fraction of the NHS's work.

If we are to make the most of our health service, we need to understand how it works and why it works that way. If we cherish its values – as surveys of public opinion consistently report – then we must understand what makes it special, so that those principles are maintained. If we want it to be better – and there is plenty of room for improvement – we need to know as much as possible about it, its origins and its development, so that we can press for the changes we want in an informed manner. This book seeks to help provide that information.

At the end of the 20th century and the beginning of the 21st, the NHS experienced a period of unprecedented innovation and upheaval for patients, clinicians, and managers. It was a period of political intrigue, controversy, and revolt; and one of realisation that general practice is the innovative and organisational powerhouse of a modern NHS. This book is a memoir, a personal account of my career from beginning to end, a career that spanned those remarkable decades. It is intentionally personal, for general practice for much of that time was a very personal, 24-hour commitment.

I try to describe the background and contemporary effect of such dramatic changes. While our practice was directly involved in several innovative projects, they were very specific. I do not promote us as something special, but rather as a single example among over 30 000 others. We were all doing similar things and, to a greater or lesser extent, in similar ways. Ours is merely the practice I knew best.

The book's different parts describe relevant elements of the history of the NHS, the training of a general practitioner (GP), the development of our general practice in terms of personnel, buildings, and information systems, and the delivery of our clinical services.

Finally, I describe several of the national projects with which we were involved, which demonstrate the growing influence of general practices on national policies.

I do not attempt to describe hospital medicine, other than through the inevitably distorted vision of a GP. There are books by authors far better qualified than I which describe that aspect of the service. But there are all too few books that describe the development of general practice, and this one contributes to addressing that gap in knowledge.

THE FIRST AND THE LAST

The first and last consultations of my career could not have been more different. Thirty-two years apart, they illustrate many of the changes that took place between them.

THE FIRST

I had qualified three years earlier and was now halfway through three years of training as a GP. I was a junior hospital doctor, but the practice at Stork House had phoned me to ask if I could help out that evening; a doctor was unwell and so away from the practice.

Number 20 Billing Road is one of a terrace of four-storey houses opposite Northampton General Hospital. It took but a moment to leave the long, impersonal corridors, with their hard lighting, harsh acoustics, and faint whiff of disinfectant to cross the road, mount the six stone steps flanked by two Victorian concrete storks and go through the door.

In the past, it had been the home of the senior partner, though he had moved out some years before to plusher accommodation. Michael Woolmore, the youngest partner, had moved in with his young family on joining the practice, but by now they had moved out too.

It still had a homely feel. Just inside the front door, on the left, a small reception hatch gave access to what would earlier have been the front parlour, but was now the combined office and waiting room. Shelves of pale fawn NHS medical records lined every wall. For patients waiting their turn, there were wooden chairs and a bench covered in rather shabby red plastic. The receptionist's desk was located by the bay window, though she met me at the hatch.

The consulting room was next along the corridor. I remember the comforting domestic style: soft tungsten lighting, pictures on the walls, and carpet on the floor. A gas fire hissed quietly in the fireplace, adding that warm, slightly damp atmosphere that only a gas fire brings. The desk was an old mahogany, kneehole affair de rigueur for doctors' consulting rooms at the time. Behind it, in the corner, stood one of those white-painted, steel and glass trolleys so typical of consulting rooms and laid out with instruments and glass bottles; a stainless-steel kidney dish contained sterilised needles and glass syringes. The epitome of a family doctor's consulting room, there were two wooden chairs for patients, one directly in front of the desk, bank manager-style, and one beside it on my right, alarmingly close to the gas fire.

The receptionist brought me a cup of tea with a biscuit in the saucer. Looking around the room, sipping my tea and downing the biscuit, I felt I had at last arrived at my personal version of AJ Cronin's *The Citadel*, no matter how unlikely the prospect had seemed to anyone aware of my academic record. It was quite a moment, though I had no idea that 18 months later the practice would become my professional home for the rest of my career.

My empty teacup pushed to one side, I started work; the very first of over 150 000 consultations I was to perform over the next 3 decades. Such a small number for a life's work, but it must be about right.

A buzzer summoned patients by sounding in the waiting room, where the receptionist gave the next patient their medical record envelope. They came along the corridor and knocked on the consulting room door, very much as one would before entering the boss's office. Sadly, in this way the patient–doctor hierarchy had been established before patients even entered the room. The doctor was king. He summoned and you went into the presence of this wise font of knowledge. You should feel lucky and grateful to be there. Interestingly, in those days patients usually did.

It was not the custom to greet patients at the door, or even to stand when they entered the room. A greeting of course, though even this was often hampered by not knowing who the patient was. Only when the record envelope was handed over, a keen eye could glimpse the name on the top.

And so my first patient came in, an 11-year-old West Indian boy accompanied by his mother. His skin was a terrible mess, with weeping, infected areas all over his body. I do not know how he could tolerate wearing clothes at all.

Severe eczema is bad enough at the best of times, but if it gets infected things can change very quickly, with the infection spreading like wildfire. Despite having worked in hospital paediatrics and dermatology, I had not seen such an infection before; it was an alarming sight. Hopefully, my slow and careful examination came across to the patient and his mother as deep professional regard, though that would be a fortunate misinterpretation.

I was flummoxed, and here was my first lesson about general practice. Not only was the GP meant to have a working knowledge of the entire compass of medicine (and much else of life besides), but they had to know what to do without reference to anyone and to be able to do it in the next minute without repetition, hesitation, or deviation. A doctor can only wash his hands for so long. More than in most areas of medicine, general practice requires an ability to think on your feet, to use and back your judgement, and always – always – to do something, no matter how simple, with conviction and reassurance.[1] In hospitals, there was always someone else to ask.

Happily, I did the right thing. I prescribed an appropriate antibiotic and asked the boy to see his doctor for review the next day. Later, I learnt that he quickly recovered with the antibiotic. As things turned out, his whole family remained lovely patients of mine for many years.

And so the consulting session moved on from patient to patient. Apart from the first boy, it was all fairly minor stuff. When it was

---

[1] Things are rather better now. It is acceptable to tell patients you want to think something over or to take advice from others; but it was not the case then, particularly if you did not know the patient.

over, I pocketed the £3 offered for my evening's work[2] and walked back across Billing Road to complete the hospital part of my GP training.

That was 1973, a very different world to how the UK is today. Few UK households had central heating, most televisions were black and white, pubs were smoky, seat belts were for rally cars and car heaters came as a pricey, optional extra. It was the year of the miners' strike and the three-day week, Watergate and America's withdrawal from Vietnam.

The practice did not use pagers, computers, or mobile phones; they had not been invented. GPs relied on phone landlines for communication, although about a fifth of our patients did not have one and had to use public telephone boxes. It was not uncommon for a doctor to return home from a night visit some miles away to find his wife waiting with the address of another patient, perhaps very near to the one he had just left.

A year after that first consultation, I finished my training and was invited to join the Billing Road partnership. There were three other doctors, two part-time receptionists, a cleaner, and her bronchitic, Woodbine-smoking[3] husband who acted as our odd-job man.

That was it. That was the practice I was joining. Between them, the partners were on call 24 hours a day, every day of the year. It was a responsibility and commitment to total care for 8500 patients.

---

[2] Equivalent to £32 in 2015, as corrected by the retail price index (RPI).
[3] Woodbine is a brand of cigarettes made in England by WD & HO Wills (now Imperial Tobacco) since 1888.

THE LAST

Things could hardly have been more different in 2006. The practice's Victorian terraced house had been replaced with a new, purpose-built medical centre, complete with its suite of nurses' treatment rooms, a large car park, a pharmacy, physiotherapist, and dentist. The tiny 1970s staff of two or three untrained, part-time receptionists had evolved into a professional primary healthcare team of practice and community nurses, managers, IT staff, receptionists, counsellors, mental health workers, a patient participation group, trainees within all disciplines, and five doctors – none of whom worked full-time within the practice. Medical records had also leapt forward from the days of Lloyd George to those of Mark Zuckerberg.

My first-floor consulting room was centrally heated, air-conditioned, and brightly lit by large windows. We all had the same basic furniture but embellished our rooms with additional furniture and items to suit us. On my walls were poster enlargements of photographs from five holidays in different countries. The game was for patients to guess the locations when they had nothing else to do, for example, if I was called away from the room.

But what of the advances in technology? The computer in a doctor's consulting room is always an intruder; all you can do is get it as right as possible. I had long learnt to point the screen halfway between patient and doctor so we could both see it. Patients would comment on my typing skills, occasionally even in complimentary tones, but more often to gently chide in amusement at my attempts to deflect a descending fingertip towards the preferred key. It all added to the sense of us working together.

Much more importantly, they could see what I was writing about them. These were their notes, not mine, so commonly we wrote them together, agreeing what I was going to type.

***

It was against that backdrop of real advances that my last patient, still in her early 50s, had come to see me 2 years previously. Let us call her Jean. Jean had shown me a lump at the top of her thigh, diagnosed by subsequent hospital tests to be a sarcoma, a malignant tumour. Jean was a stoic. She refused to give up her effervescent enthusiasm for life, even during the traumas of two local excisions, chemotherapy, radiotherapy, recurrences, and ultimately a major, hindquarter amputation of her leg through the hip joint. After each of these therapeutic assaults, she would gather herself once more and move on with her life, even when reduced to swinging along with two sticks and one leg in her usual frenetic hurry, head down in concentration. Not a moment of life was to be wasted; her clock was ticking faster than most.

Eventually, she came to see me again with bad news. She had been to the hospital the day before to be told that, despite all therapeutic efforts, her tumour had spread further and was now untreatable. There was nothing more to be done. She was terminal, and she knew it.

For a while, Jean carried on at home with support from the local Cynthia Spencer Hospice,[4] but eventually she needed admission there. I visited her about a week before I retired. She was her usual inspirational self, and we chatted for a while about nothing in particular. It was then I decided to visit her again on my last day in practice, to make her the last consultation of my career.

On the morning of my retirement, I drove out to the hospice where the staff told me she was now so ill that she was in the special area for those close to death. She was refusing all visitors, but they had a word and I was invited along to see her. We had a lovely conversation. I suppose it was the ultimate opportunity; neither patient nor doctor had anything to lose at all; it was the end for both of us, albeit in very different ways. We talked for a short while, and then we said our goodbyes. I was profoundly sad about the loss of a wonderful

---

[4] Cynthia Spencer Hospice provides specialist palliative care services for South Northamptonshire.

personality, clear in thought to the end but let down by her failing physical support system. I had a deep satisfaction at such a final moment in my career as a personal doctor. It was the perfect way to drop the curtain.

The next day the practice put on an evening retirement party for me, and it was there that one of the partners told me Jean had died that morning.

***

Much had changed in the 34 years between that first consultation at the Billing Road surgery and the last one, at the hospice. It was a time of unprecedented innovation and change in the NHS, particularly in general practice, and I was fortunate to be a GP throughout that era.

PART ONE

IN THE BEGINNING

Part One sets the scene for the book. It describes what it was like to be a medical student and young doctor in the second half of the 1960s and early 1970s, and it gives the background of my practice. It also offers a personal perspective of what it is like to be seriously ill.

THE DOCTOR'S TALE

DECISIONS, DECISIONS, DECISIONS

How and why do we choose a career? Or indeed any use of our time? Perhaps it follows considered analysis, with or without the influence of others. Perhaps it is indirect; we sway like flotsam with the changing tides of circumstance and fortune until we settle on some suitable shore.

My decision fell into the camp of a considered analysis, though its actual realisation owed a great deal to good fortune. Like many other four-year-olds, I was already considering my career options with earnest intent. For example, I could not be a firefighter, much as I would love to ride on the fire engine and squirt water, because there would be a distinct risk of getting burnt. Sadly, that one was struck from the list.

Continuing with the predilection for uniforms so typical of that age, I considered joining the police force. Again, this had a lot of attractions, including the ownership of a pair of handcuffs, but – to be weighed against that – was the possibility of personal injury. Another rejection. Of course, there was the army, but by now you will follow my thoughts on that one.

My mother had been a nurse and did kind, "nursey" things whenever I grazed my knees, or had a cough or toothache. Of course, that is normal behaviour for a mother, but somehow in my eyes her previous career also received credit. Then again, our family doctor was a nice man. Dr Barwood came and sat on my bed when I was poorly (doctors did that in the 1950s), took his time, and was kind to me. What intrigued me most about him was that while he used his stethoscope to listen to the front of my chest, he threw his head back, closed his eyes in concentration, and breathed through his open mouth, thus providing me with a clear view up his nose. I know now why he did it (you can hear better through the stethoscope), but it seemed odd at the time.

Unlike all the other careers on my shortlist, I could not think of anything against being a doctor. There were no baddies to hurt me, no fires to burn me, and I would not drown – the issue that had drawn a line through the otherwise attractive lifeboat service. And so, the decision was made. Surprisingly, I never changed my mind. Not for a moment. So, six decades later, when Tadiwa, my grandson in Zimbabwe who was three years old at the time, earnestly told me his plans I listened respectfully, though I confess to finding his aspiration to be a cheetah unrealistic. Then again, I expect that is exactly what adults said about me when I was his age!

Despite a school record distinguished by woeful lassitude, I managed to "hedge-hop" the required academic barriers and, in October 1965, began training at the Middlesex Hospital Medical School in central London. Naturally, this surprised every teacher who had ever known me, but pleasingly it achieved the ambition of a four-year-old. I fear Tadiwa will find the fulfilment of his dream an even sterner task, but naturally, I wish him well.

MEDICAL SCHOOL

Medical school in the 1960s was unlike most other university courses. Perhaps it still is. It was a five-year vocational training; an apprenticeship rather than an academic education. For the 18 months of preclinical studies, we had lectures from 9 a.m. until 5 p.m., 5 days a week. There were frequent assessments and work to do most evenings. It was slightly more grown-up than the sixth form,[5] but not much.

---

[5] In the UK, this is the two final years at school for students between the ages of 16 and 18 who are preparing for A or AS level public exams.

We sat in tiered lecture theatres where – down at the front – fearsome professors paced. They scared the living daylights out of me, and I kept as far away from them as possible. There, too, were a couple of rows of the very keenest and, it has to be said, brightest students – one of whom I was to marry. Conversely, my rowing friends and I sat up at the back, near the door, where we could more easily slip into our seats when late for lectures, perhaps with a half-eaten slice of breakfast toast still in hand.

There was an enormous amount of information to assimilate: physiology, genetics, histology, biochemistry, and anatomy, the latter taught in far greater detail than is now deemed necessary. We had real bodies to dissect in those days. The top floor's dissecting room was a large rectangular space: white walls, high ceiling, bright lighting illuminating two rows of carefully arranged, stainless-steel mortuary tables, and all gently suffused with the sickly sweet, cloying smell of formaldehyde preservative.

It was a sombre place, though by no means macabre. Lecturers and students all wore white coats, with the usual undergraduate banter now subdued. The only person in a dark suit was the tall, Twiggy-thin,[6] very Scottish professor of anatomy. Terrifying. Professor Walls moved silently, stealthily between the dissecting tables, cocking his head from side to side to peer with gimlet eye at whatever we were doing. A heron, stalking its prey.

Despite the infamous jocularity of medical students at that time, within the dissecting room we had a very real respect for the 10 people before us who had donated their bodies to the study of medicine. We were divided into groups of 6 or so, and a body allocated to each for the duration of the 18-month preclinical course. The medical schools treated bodies with great propriety and

---

[6] Twiggy is the pseudonym of Lesley Hornby, an English model, actress, and singer. A British cultural icon, she was a prominent teenage model in 1960s London.

afterwards returned them with due ceremony to their next of kin for burial.

It is different now. For one thing, it makes perfect sense for anatomy to be taught in far less mind-numbing detail, detail that served no purpose whatsoever in most of our careers. Now students use plastic models and computer graphics rather than cadavers. Professor Walls must be turning in his grave.

After 18 months, we could enter clinical studies, provided we passed the dreaded 2nd MB examination.[7] It was a period of concentrated study far removed from the traditional perception of university life; in some ways, it was more an exercise in memory than a training of lasting practical benefit. Along with law exams, it was regarded at the time as the hardest challenge to confront any British university undergraduate. You could resit 2nd MB once, but fail it twice and you were out of medical school for good.

During our clinical studies, we wore half-length white coats stuffed with pens, aides-memoires, notes, and shiny new stethoscopes. Divided into "firms" of eight students, we rotated through different specialities, each lasting a few months. By this means, we experienced all the required hospital disciplines before the end of our three and a half years of clinical training.

Life on the wards was a welcome change from the pressure of preclinical studies. It was more relevant and exciting, there was a pleasant, measured pace, and we were treated as adults and postgraduates rather than schoolchildren. We had left the university lecture room. We were now members of the hospital community, albeit very much at the bottom of the food chain.

On each firm, we were allocated a small number of patients. We

---

[7] The University of London medical degree is still the MBBS, Bachelor of Medicine, Bachelor of Surgery. At that time, there were three major exams: you could be exempt from 1st MB by having suitable science A levels; 2nd MB was taken after 18 months of preclinical studies; and finals was the third phase, taken after a further three and a half years of clinical studies.

made up the initial set of medical records on the patient's admission, took blood samples each morning, organised X-rays, and so on. We also attended *Doctor in the House*-style ward rounds,[8] trailing around in loose formation behind specialists who were seemingly the only ones to enjoy the occasion. I am sure the patients did not.

Despite any weaknesses, the medical school of the 1960s was a reasonable apprenticeship-style training, and the patients were both understanding and kind. Some would even offer conspiratorial help when being the case studies at exam time. A fellow student found the whispered "Have you examined my liver yet, doctor?" a most helpful nudge!

PAYING FOR UNIVERSITY

The funding of going to university was very different in the early 1970s. First, it was free of all tuition fees. On top of that, thanks to the Education Act 1962, every student was entitled to a maintenance grant, means-tested against the parents' income. There was no such thing as a subsidised student loan either; the Student Loan Company did not come into existence until 1990. In effect, we were being paid for going to university. At the time, we did not realise how lucky we were; we do now.

OFF DUTY

But there is more to university than just study, and any student will have numerous stories of college days. The following is one of the most remarkable of mine.

---

[8] Richard Gordon (pen name of Gordon Ostlere, an English surgeon and anaesthetist) is best-known for writing a long series of comic novels on a medical theme beginning with *Doctor in the House*, which were subsequently adapted for film, television, radio, and the stage.

My interests revolved around rowing, woodwork, and hi-fi. I had built loudspeakers before, but a new pair was, of course, to be bigger and better. A magazine described cylindrical speaker cabinets, pointing out that a cylinder cannot vibrate as readily as the more usual rectangular box, and so the bass frequencies would be less distorted.

Students, like most young people, enjoy bass and this sounded like a good idea. I reasoned that the more solid the cylinder, the better. I visited a builder's yard and bought two concrete sewer pipes. I bolted the loudspeaker unit to a thick plywood base and fixed it into the concrete pipe with glass fibre resin. Finally, I mounted an inverted aluminium cone above each to deflect the sound out to the sides from the upward-facing speakers and built sturdy wooden trolleys on castors for them. The sound they produced was staggering. For sure they did not vibrate, but everything else did!

I had just moved into the third floor of the brand-new Astor College in Charlotte Street, a hall of residence built under the auspices of Lord Astor specifically for Middlesex Hospital students. One afternoon an odd thing happened. I was having a short siesta in my room, as students do, when there was a knock on the door. I opened it to find the rather serious college administrator outside. She introduced her companion, the head builder; there was still some final work going on elsewhere in the college.

"We understand you have some big loudspeakers in here," one of them said. I was delighted to show off my creations, even if surprised at this unexpected interest, and somewhat embarrassed to be dressed only in a towel hastily wrapped around my waist. But there was a concern too: the college rules only permitted a "small music system" in one's room. As I showed them in, I enquired about the problem.

"The problem is in the next room," one of them said. So, we all trooped into the corridor to look in the next room, which was still unoccupied. On the party wall shared with my room, a large area of plaster had come away from the wall, up to about a metre from the floor and about half way along it. It was as if someone had cut the plaster horizontally with a Stanley knife, in a dead straight line, right through to the plasterboard, so that the plaster fell to the floor below it. I had never seen anything like it and have not since.

"We think your speakers did this."

"How on earth could that have happened?" I responded, desperately trying to think things through while being only too aware that my student's grant would not run to paying for building repairs.

We went back to my room to study Tom and Jerry, the two speakers standing defiantly on the opposite side of the offending party wall. It was abundantly clear to me that the horizontal line on the opposite side of the party wall was at precisely the same level as the top of the aluminium diffusers on my loudspeakers, placed there for the express purpose of deflecting sound waves horizontally.

"Do they move?" they asked, suspiciously eyeing the plinths beneath each speaker.

"Absolutely. They are on castors." I judged it best to sound unconcerned.

At this point, they were dusted by my guardian angel and deprived of their senses. A glint of conviction appeared in their eyes. "Then it seems you have rolled one of the speakers across your room and hit the wall, knocking the plaster off the other side."

I was momentarily lost for words, but you must take the opportunities life offers. "OK, so if that is what happened, then surely there will at least be a dent in my wall where it struck."

It seemed a logical supposition, so we all gathered around to peer at my wall, with me desperately clutching at my ever-loosening towel. Fortunately, the wall was dent-free, which threw them. After a few more stressful moments they took their leave, agreeing that there must be some other explanation for this most remarkable incident. "Perhaps a faulty plaster mix?" I offered, as I bid them farewell.

Closing the door, I adjusted my towel and sat down on the edge of the bed in a state of shaking, stunned relief. As I did so, I noticed a pair of green, women's shoes poking out from under the bed, forgotten in the confusion as the administrator knocked on the door.

I stood up and opened the wardrobe door.

***

We got married in our final year. Some politicians would ruefully confirm that it is not easy to keep a relationship secret for two years in a closed community. But we wanted to do so and did. Eventually, we went public and became engaged halfway through our clinical studies, pleasingly to most people's complete surprise. A year later, I took my final exams and qualified as a doctor. The whole of medicine now lay before me.

THE PATIENT'S TALE

It can help a doctor to have been seriously ill. They gain an insight into what it is like to be on the other side of the desk, to experience kindness or a lack of empathy, delay or quick access, fear and reassurance.

I can foresee that within future medical training, the use of virtual reality technologies will allow such simulation, and perhaps that is a practical way forward. If our purpose is to provide a caring service to patients, it is useful to have been one. At least, that is my experience.

***

It was a beautiful late winter morning, and while visiting an older patient, I noticed that by looking out of her bedroom window I could see right across the broad Nene Valley to my new house a couple of miles away. Except I seemed to have two, one slightly on top of the other. Suddenly I felt faint; my legs gave way and I sat down very quickly on the side of the bed, which handily was just behind me.

This was not as alarming for the lady as you might think, as she was unconscious. She had suffered a major stroke a couple of days before and, before the times and benefits of specialist stroke units, was now peacefully slipping away exactly where she would have wanted to be, in her bed. Her daughter had left the room to fetch something and, lacking anyone to talk to, I was enjoying the view from her window. By the time the daughter returned I had collected myself, turned to face her mother, and was no doubt looking suitably concerned. Who I was concerned about at that precise moment was, I hope, far less obvious.

As soon as I finished my visiting round, I phoned a specialist friend. I felt unable to go to my GP because the root of the problem was clearly work-related stress, and he was one of my partners. That would be embarrassing for both of us.

The specialist suggested I saw him that afternoon, in my tea break. Perfect. I was fully booked that afternoon but had a 20-minute break, and the hospital was just across the road from our surgery. During my tea break, I nipped across the road to see him.

His assessment was that I had a tumour in the back of my brain, probably an acoustic neuroma. Not stress after all, then. What was more, it must have been quite large, as there were haemorrhages at the back of my eyes caused by raised pressure within my skull.

This completely unexpected news came as a bit of a blow. I left the hospital in a daze, crossed the road and continued with the second half of my consulting session. Naturally, the first patient I saw was complaining of headaches.

So, the first lesson is that the blindingly obvious can elude the individual concerned. It seems incredible that I had such little self-awareness, but similar stories are not uncommon. Sometimes, in all sorts of situations, what should be glaringly obvious is somehow opaque.

***

Being admitted to hospital for investigations is strange, particularly if you feel well. Suddenly you are captive to the schedules of others. Medicine is like that. Consider its use of patronising and commanding verbs, behaviour albeit less pronounced now than in the past. "I will refer you to the hospital." From there we are "allowed to go home" by being "discharged", someone no longer required nor wanted. This is one human trying to help another.

Perhaps we are not even warned that some investigation or other is going to happen until the kindly porter comes with his wheelchair or trolley, our tumbril to the gallows. We feel out of control, a sack on a conveyor belt. And when we get there, a process begins. An instruction to lie on a metal table. Are you allergic to iodine? You do not think so, which is apparently good enough. You did not say "Yes", so it is one for the "No" box. Tick. They did ask. Earplugs in. The radiographer explains the need to lie still. Dye injected into a vein; cold feeling up your arm. Electric motors glide you into a narrow, cylindrical tunnel. Only just room all round. Try to see the funny side.

"Are you OK in there?" Nice voice. Footsteps receding, a door shuts. Silence. Utter silence.

What now? More reassurance and explanation, this time over an intercom inside the tunnel. Then, a few staccato clicks followed by the noise they warned you about: throbbing, rhythmical sounds, whooshing around your head like a pulse. It is loud; earplugs were a good idea. Health and safety no doubt. Patient wearing earplugs? Tick.

Lie very still. Nod big toe in time to the whooshing rhythm to distract from the closed-in feeling. Hope moving toe is OK. They said lie still, but the toe is not even in the contraption, and they are scanning your head, not a foot. Carry on. Anarchy feels good.

Tickly nose coming on. Ah! Arms trapped by side. What happens if I sneeze? Try not to. Keep head still and concentrate on toe. Tickle recedes.

All suddenly quiet. A door opens, footsteps coming closer.

"All done!"

Motorised regurgitation from the tunnel and help getting off the bed; pushed back to the ward in another chair. You feel you should be looking ill if you need all this transport. Perhaps you do. There is a thought!

The ward now feels safe and home. "OK mate?" asks the cheery cockney in the next bed. It is lunchtime.

In the afternoon, another trip in a wheelchair. A special test, apparently. See the funny side to keep up morale – you would pay for trips like this at a funfair. Odd to be pushed along facing everyone, waist high; a child's view once more. You had not realised how embarrassing it is. People gawp, discretely. What has he got? What indeed?

The senior registrar greets you again, this time in a funny little room in the basement bowels of the hospital. You lie on your left side as instructed, right ear aimed at the ceiling, defenceless, apprehensive, waiting. Everything is fine until he tries to be modern and helpful. "This is a specialised hearing test. I want you to keep very still for me; I am just going to push a needle through your eardrum."

Now, there are times in life when it is better not to know exactly what is going to happen to you. This is one of them. Fear paralyses you. Just as well; thrashing around is a bad idea.

In fact, it is not too bad at all, any physical discomfort failing to compete with the terror engendered by the thought of a needle probing around those three tiny bones we struggle to remember in *Trivial Pursuit* – the malleus, incus, and the other one. Maybe the doctor is using cocaine. Not personally, you understand, but as an anaesthetic in your ear. If so, it works.

And so, eventually, back to the ward, and my cheery cockney companion. Thank heavens for public wards. There is comfort in company.

By the following evening, the investigations are finished. The specialist comes to tell you the results in quiet, practical tones. It is long after most senior staff have gone home, and there is none of the fawning entourage on which most consultants thrive. He sits on the side of the bed, conveying important messages in just the right way. Consulting.

The next morning the nurses say you can go home. Discharged. Collect your clothes, do not pass *Go*, do not collect £200. The hospital will contact you in a few weeks when they have a bed for your operation.

You go home and wonder how you get ready for brain surgery.

Swimming seems a good idea; presumably, the fitter you are the better. Off work, so swimming every morning makes a surprising difference in a couple of weeks. Suddenly people seem to be taking an awful lot of photographs of you, but the attention is nice.

Back in the hospital, a few weeks later, you are treated to a free haircut, in bed. Another new experience. The barber, brisk but kindly, even offers a choice of styles. All or half? He only has to shave the right, but he advises most prefer it all off. Otherwise, it looks a bit funny. You take his advice and opt for the house special, the "total". He approves.

You sleep, surprisingly, and are gently woken by a nurse shortly after 5 a.m. It is time to start getting ready for your operation. You miss your breakfast like never before – we always want what we cannot have – but enjoy wallowing in a deep hot bath of soapy disinfectant. Now dressed in your risqué, backless theatre gown you sheepishly return to your bed to await events.

The staff nurse comes to give the pre-med injection, and you ask the obvious. "Will the operation be delayed?"

"Don't worry. That won't happen. They have booked the operating theatre from 8 a.m. for you. For the whole day."

For the whole day? You are still mulling over that comment when you drift off into a dry-mouthed tranquillity.

You must have got to the anaesthetic room somehow, but have no memory of the tumbril. The clock over the door of the anaesthetic room says exactly eight o'clock, and you think how efficient everyone is to start on time. Or was that a dream – there is no way of knowing – but it is a vivid image to this day.

Then, immediately, like a snap of the fingers, you are somewhere completely different. There is no sensation of going to sleep, not even of feeling sleepy or closing your eyes, nor of waking up. Over 36 hours have passed, and you are in the hospital's intensive care unit (ICU), barely awake and with a dry mouth.

You ask a charge nurse if you can suck an ice cube. Of course, you cannot, but no drink has been as glorious as the iced water that is carefully trickled into your mouth a few minutes later. You will remember that simple act of kindness all your life.

You feel awful. You while away a few moments trying to work out how many tubes they have stuck into you. You give up at seven, or is it six? Oh, what the hell!

The operation had gone on until 1 a.m. in the morning, but even then they had not been able to remove the whole thing. Acoustic neuromas are usually tiny, a pea or broad bean, but this was a very juicy satsuma measuring 7–8 cm in diameter. You are told it will take a second operation to finish the job, this time sneaking up behind it from another direction. Another hole in your head; you will end up with a skull like a colander. So, a week later everyone goes back to the operating theatre for round two, and the job is done.

Or, at least the surgery is done. But on the ward, neurosurgical observations are a handy introduction to torture. Every 15 minutes, day and night, a nurse comes to ask you questions to check that you are alive, and that as far as can be judged you will remain so until their next visit. This is no problem during the day, but at night it becomes quite irksome.

Always the same questions; always the same answers. Unless you are feeling particularly weary and obtuse, when purposely giving the wrong answer provides slight satisfaction.

"Who is the prime minister?"

"I didn't know we had one."

"Where are you?"

"The same place as you."

They are kind and understanding, and seem to excuse the anger, swearing, and deliberately evasive answers.

After a few days, the frequency goes down to half hourly, then hourly. Presumably, the chance of death within a given amount of time is judged to be receding, which you consider encouraging.

The doctors and nurses come across as being wonderful, demonstrating enormous skill, empathy, and dedication. You learn once and for all the depth of trust a patient can develop for a clinician, and the additional therapeutic benefit accruing from that trust. Comments such as "If patients are really ill they will be glad to see anyone" are facile and just plain wrong. It is when patients are very ill that they most need to see a clinician whom they trust. Ask any hospice.

In many ways, you become very childlike in a hospital; you are dependent on others, with no responsibilities or discretion of your own. Being ill can remove the pressure to work, go to school, or do any number of things we may not want to do. So, some will welcome the sick role, but for others the opposite applies, and they become frustrated at the shackles their illness puts on them. Every day GPs witness both points of view.

Hospital staff act *in loco parentis*. Perhaps that is why patients can be so furious when the medical world fails them. They felt entitled to trust it and it had betrayed that trust. My team (we patients always own our clinical advisers, as in "my doctor", "my nurse", "my dentist", "my proctologist") were simply incapable of doing anything at all that was not perfection itself.

Nurses, doctors, porters – my faith in all of them would have done a Labrador proud. The ward cleaner was a gem; they usually are. She brought me a cup of tea in the morning, chatted away as she mopped around the room, and later came with the paper trolley, which happily also stocked Nutty Bars. Of course, her duties did not include the disquieting lumbar punctures, injections, neurological observations, and dressing changes. It was not for her to bring the unexpected porter's tumbril, perhaps to carry you off to some new discomfort.

You could relax, have a chat, joke, or buy a paper. She was safe; she did you good.

Eventually, it is time to go home, an excitement and release so intense you cannot sleep the night before – unlike even the night before brain surgery – and the morning rituals now drag in their suddenly diminished importance. No doctors about, but that is usually the case. The nurses are pleased for you. They wish you well, a speedy recovery, come back and see us; and then, of course, they turn to get on. You have been discharged and they have work to do.

Once home, your team changes again. Now it is the GP and district nurses, but mainly your family, who take the strain. You convalesce at home for much longer than you were in hospital – three weeks there, but three months at home. You are weak but well. Brain surgery can be unusual in that way. No soreness. No pain at all; the brain may know what pain is everywhere else, but has no pain receptors of its own.[9] You are just waiting; waiting to recover.

Eventually, even the convalescence is over and you return to work. It is strange for your colleagues. Will he cope? Will we have to step in and cover him? Is he OK clinically? Sensible and understandable questions. None of us knew the answers. And it is strange for patients too, most of whom are well aware that you have been seriously ill. Some have exaggerated ideas of its gravity and treat you as if you will be away again soon, perhaps for good. But all show a touching concern. Slowly all these things fade. Life returns to normal; everyone moves on, and that is the end of that.

***

Why does this matter here? It matters because, ultimately, healthcare is not just about hospitals, clinical commissioning groups

---

[9] In contrast, the meninges, the membranes lining the outside of the brain, are very pain sensitive, as experienced by anyone with meningitis or raised intracranial pressure.

(CCGs), evidence-based medicine, general practice, pharmacy, or dentistry. It is about individual people. It is important because the art of medicine matters as well as the science. The neurosurgeon who treated me was a world authority on my condition, but he was also a quiet, dedicated, empathic physician. He knew instinctively how to communicate with his patients, so gaining their immediate trust.

My experience demonstrated the kindness and professionalism of NHS staff. I learnt a great deal about human relationships; that no matter how many flashing lights and whirring machines there are, it is the empathic, maternal things that impact most on patients, such as kindness, warmth, gentleness, and the perception of undivided, empathic attention. A sip of iced water from someone who understood. The archetypal soldier dying on a battlefield cries out not for a surgeon, but for his mother. As Ann Cartwright had observed a few years earlier, patients take clinical expertise for granted; it is these softer matters they look for.[10]

In some ways, I am glad I was ill, but I was lucky. Other than a few neurological sequelae, I made a full recovery thanks to the nature of the problem itself and the availability of excellent care. Sadly, fate was less kind to many of my patients, but I hope my experience helped me help them more than if I had not been through it myself.

---

[10] Cartwright A, Anderson R (1979). *Patients and Their Doctors 1977. Report on Some Changes in General Practice Between 1964 and 1977 for the Royal Commission on the National Health Service.* London, Royal College of General Practitioners.

THE PRACTICE'S TALE

My senior partner Christopher Elliott-Binns wrote a book about the practice, and I am grateful to its publishers for letting me use it as a resource for this chapter.

***

We can begin in 1844, when Queen Victoria passed through Northampton by rail on her way from London to Burghley House, a magnificent Elizabethan mansion at Stamford, Lincolnshire. Seizing the opportunity, the elders of Northampton arranged for the royal pause to become an official visit rather than just a comfort break at the station.

Clearly, the Victorians took such a royal visit very seriously indeed. To mark the occasion, a public subscription in the town raised £1300[11] to build Corinth House, the "Royal Victoria Dispensary". A handsome white building, it looked vaguely like a much smaller version of the White House in Washington DC, built 50 years earlier. Situated in Albion Place, just off Derngate in the centre of town, Corinth House played an interesting part in the local medical life before being demolished in 1960 to make way for a municipal car park.

It is worth noting the Dispensary's declared purpose in 1845:

> *To enable families efficient medical advice and medicine during illness by their own, small periodic payments, with assistance of contributions from the more opulent.*[12]

---

[11] Adjusted in line with average earnings, £1300 in 1834 equated to just over £1 million in 2014.

[12] Elliott-Binns C (1992). *The Story of a Northampton Practice 1845–1992*. Northampton, Aster Print, p. 11.

That was very early for such broad-minded, societal thoughts concerning medicine, welfare, and addressing inequalities. The Poor Law Amendment Act 1834 was only 10 years old, and the National Insurance Act was 67 years distant. It would be a century before the NHS came into being.

The cost of being part of the Dispensary's high-minded programme was a penny a week for adults, a halfpenny for children or 2 pence[13] for the whole family. Patients had to provide their own bottles for medicine, midwifery services cost a remarkably modest 5 shillings all in,[14] but vaccinations were free, as indeed they were at the town's hospital, reflecting the value put on the prevention of infectious diseases.

Christopher's book claims the Royal Victoria Dispensary was our earliest building, but he does not suggest it was ours exclusively. In fact, we cannot be sure of our involvement at the very beginning at all. But we do know that in 1847, three years later, our Dr Branwhite Spurgin was one of its medical officers, remaining on the staff for 22 years. He may well have been there at the start. After that, his place at the Dispensary was taken by Dr William Barr, his successor in our practice. By 1890, there were six doctors on the staff, of which two were from our practice. On such slender threads hangs our claim to major association!

In retrospect, what is most interesting is that when Christopher wrote his book in the 1980s, we wanted that historical link. The practice was our life, we were committed to it, proud of it, and wanted to know from where it had come.

There are benefits in that archival interest. For example, we can get a glimpse of a doctor's workload at the end of the 19th century from the records of the Royal Victoria Dispensary. During 1880, William Barr conducted 11 354 consultations at either Corinth House or his

---

[13] This corresponded to £0.74 per week in 2014, if inflated by the RPI.
[14] This corresponded to £22.30 in 2014, if inflated by the RPI.

home, and an additional 13 640 house calls: a total of 24 994 consultations, or about 520 per working week. Exactly 100 years later and in the same practice, my total was 5469 for the year, or 118 per week. Home visits made up 55% of Dr Barr's workload, while they were a mere 15% of mine. And by the end of my career, home visits had receded still further, to under 5% of my workload. Now, a further 10 years on, they would be much lower again.

Of course, consultations in 1880 were very different to how they are now, often consisting of a quick word, a glance at the tongue, and the issuing of a prescription for coloured medicine. GPs became masters of the snap diagnosis. Most of the benefit of seeing a doctor arose from the occasion; later we shall see how the doctor himself was the primary therapeutic agent. The available drugs were of little value, and occasionally harmful, so a GP had to employ other skills: giving comfort and reassurance, exuding a Victorian air of professional competence, and offering wisdom and precise, dogmatic instruction as to what should, and should not, be done. By such authoritative methods, GPs calmed anxiety and reassured the patient, giving the natural healing process time to take place, and perhaps even helping it along.

The Royal Victoria Dispensary was a great success and for 75 years provided reasonable, devoted care to the town's poor. As a system of collective, population-based medical care it was ahead of national developments, and a foretaste of what was to follow, the National Insurance Act 1911. Perversely, the services instigated by that Act replaced much that was offered by the Dispensary, and not long afterwards it closed, its pioneering job done.

But its memory remained. One morning in 2005, I recognised Corinth House in a painting hanging over the fireplace in the house of an older patient; I had seen a photo of it in Christopher's book.

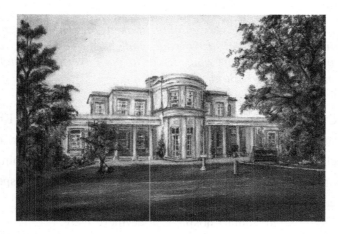

Corinth House as painted by a patient and hanging over her fireplace.

Apparently, the lady's father had bought the building as a family home when the Dispensary closed in the 1920s. She had painted the picture herself, and pointed out the window of the first-floor bedroom in which she was born! She let me borrow it to photograph, and when I retired, I gave a coloured print of it to the practice.

***

William Barr, he of the jaw-dropping 1880 workload, had an eventful career before he came to the practice. During the Crimean War, he volunteered for duty as a military staff assistant surgeon and travelled by sea to Scutari (now Üsküdar), a district of Istanbul on the Asian shore of the Bosphorus. On arrival, he was posted to the Barrack Hospital, where Florence Nightingale was already hard at work. Reports describe a nightmare, with between 2000 and 4000 troops and officers treated in appalling circumstances. One report states that there were 12 chamber pots for the entire hospital. Given that the overwhelming majority of cases were of gastroenteritis and dysentery, no elaboration is required concerning the conditions for patients. According to William Barr's diary, he was responsible for about 100 of them at any one time. He wrote:

Miss Nightingale is very highly spoken of. The kitchen is invaluable. Sago and arrowroot can be procured for any number in a very short time, while in the government kitchen you might have to wait for eternity.[15]

In the Crimean War, there were 251 200 deaths among the Russian, Bulgarian, French, and British forces, of which 15% were on the battlefield, 15% died later from their wounds, but an astonishing 70% were from disease. Of those, most were from dysentery or unspecified diarrhoea.

For example, at Scutari hospital alone there were 122 deaths over 3 days in the middle of January 1855, a month that also saw the deaths of 7 doctors and 3 nurses. But by June, after just months of Florence Nightingale's kitchen, and the work of her nurses on the wards, the monthly death toll had plummeted to single figures, a quite remarkable, personal contribution to the saving of lives.

At the end of the war, William Barr left the Crimea, returned to England, and joined Dr Branwhite Spurgin in our practice at both 55 Sheep Street and the Royal Victoria Dispensary.

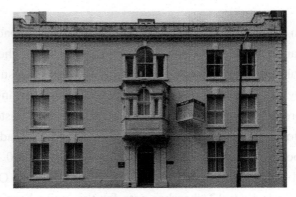

55 Sheep Street, Northampton, today.
Photograph © by Michael Sobanja.

---

[15] Elliott-Binns C (1992). *The Story of a Northampton Practice 1845–1992.* Northampton, Aster Print, p. 18.

The building in Sheep Street still stands, a grand, terraced façade. Branwhite Spurgin, at least, was far from poor.

And so, the practice's history goes on through the different doctors who worked there. The wondrously named Robert Bradley Roe served as a surgeon at the Battle of the Somme in 1916. Repatriated after collapsing from operating for 72 hours without a break, he recovered and went back to the Somme for further service. After the war, he joined the practice, and in 1928 moved to live at 20 Billing Road, converting the stable at the bottom of the garden into a surgery. It remained the practice's official premises until 1962.

He was said to have a wonderful bedside manner; when I joined the practice, older patients would recall how they felt better as soon as he entered the room. In his book, Christopher recounts a particularly charming story about Bradley Roe. It is worth repeating here because – although it may seem romantic now, idealised, and extreme – it is nonetheless true, and it encapsulates much about the best of family practice at that time, and perhaps not a little about how things have changed.

One lady had belonged to a different practice when she had her first baby, a boy born prematurely. His condition was critical and when she asked her doctor what she should do, he looked at the inert baby and remarked: "Let sleeping dogs lie."

This was hardly tactful and she changed practice to Dr Bradley Roe. He took enormous care of the baby and obtained lactalbumin, an artificial feed made by a Dutch firm and costing three shillings and six pence for a tiny jar, for him. Although this was very expensive he never charged her for it.

She had gone to him as a paying patient and the final bill was for £5 two shillings and sixpence. She told him she could not afford this and he said: "All right, then. You keep the £5 and I'll take the two and six pence."[16]

Dr Jim Mitchell was the senior partner when I arrived in 1975. He was another war veteran, captured by the Japanese after the fall of Singapore. He spent three years in the notorious Changi prison, working as the assistant surgeon in the hospital. Conditions were dreadful. He operated on cases such as perforated ulcers and appendicitis using a table in the quartermaster's stores, with instruments sterilised in the camp's kitchen boiler. There is no record of what anaesthetics, if any, were available to him. After his release, he returned to the UK weighing a mere 60 kg from starvation (he was a big man), and his skin and eyes yellow from the antimalarial drugs given after his release.

Eventually, he went into practice with Robert Bradley Roe in the converted stable at the back of 20 Billing Road. There they worked together until Bradley Roe retired in 1955, to be replaced by Christopher Elliott-Binns.

Christopher was the first to have undertaken any formal training in general practice. He had been an assistant to a single-handed practitioner in Bletchley, Buckinghamshire, though that bore little resemblance to the structured training schemes of today. He told many hair-raising stories about his early days in training, including how he carried out a successful breech delivery in a narrowboat moored on the canal, the only flickering illumination being from a gas lamp.

***

---

[16] Elliott-Binns C (1992). *The Story of a Northampton Practice 1845–1992.* Northampton, Aster Print, p. 29.

In the late 1950s, the work at Billing Road consisted solely of surgeries and visits. It was devoid of the administration and other distractions that now assail GPs. Morning surgery was from 8:30 to 9:30 a.m., and evening surgery from 6:00 to 8:00 p.m. All consulting sessions tended to run late because of uncontrolled demand and the lack of an appointment system. Any number of patients could turn up, and all were seen. The doctors visited obsessively. They had a ledger of older patients whom they visited every month. The process was largely nonsense, as these patients were often fit enough to go shopping in town. Much later, Christopher commented that looking back, it all seemed a dreadful waste of time.

In his book, Christopher sketches a picture of general practice in Northampton in the 1950s. Competition for patients caused serious animosity; doctors from different practices would not speak to one another and even crossed the street to avoid each other. Postgraduate education for GPs was almost non-existent, consisting of the odd lecture in which specialists – most of whom had never done a day's general practice in their lives – told them how to do their job.

In 1955, he worked in the converted stable at 20 Billing Road, where he had to heat water in the steriliser to wash his hands, and then transfer it to the basin "in a green enamel mug kept especially for the purpose". His consulting cubicle was miniscule, probably a horse's stall in dimension, and as the jammed window would not open, it became unbearably hot in the summer.

There was still no appointment system; in fact, little had changed in working practice since Victorian days. Christopher always felt that their giant leap forward was the purchase of two date stamps, one for Jim Mitchell and one for himself. It was some years before they bought a typewriter, though that came to a sticky end when their new partner, Michael Woolmore, backed his car over it on his first day in the practice.[17]

---

[17] I never had the courage to ask why the typewriter was in the road.

Michael and his wife Amelia arrived in 1964, complete with two small children and a third on the way. By now the surgery had moved from the stable into two floors of the house, so there was ample room for the Woolmores to live on the other two floors until they found a home of their own.

The arrangement was not quite as convenient as might appear. Their living quarters were in the basement of the house, yet their bedrooms were on the top floor of what was a four-storey house. The practice and its patients used the two floors in between. Michael and Amelia still recall the 59 steps between their kitchen and living room in the basement, and the top floor containing their bedrooms. There was no basin or toilet in the basement, and worse, there was none on the top floor either. At 6:00 p.m. every evening, patients waiting on the landing outside the first-floor consulting rooms were treated to a sequence of dressing-gowned little Woolmores coming down stairs from the top floor to brush their teeth in the bathroom beside the waiting area.

The next year, 1965, saw the publication of the *Charter for the Family Doctor Service*, in terms of long-term effect still the most important document in the history of NHS general practice.[18] It was to initiate the dawn of modern general practice. Doctors viewed the attachment of a district nurse and health visitor with mixed feelings, but found the arrangement worked well. The nurses improved the care of infants, their mothers, and patients confined to their homes. No one realised it for some years, but the practice's clinical team had been born.

The end of the 1960s also brought a significant administrative innovation: the introduction of an appointment system. Evening surgeries were now more organised; they began earlier and finished by about six o'clock. At the same time, doctors started sharing night and weekend duties with two other single-handed practices. The first green

---

[18] See "The Four Cornerstones" chapter in Part Two for more on the Charter.

shoots of organisation were emerging, accompanied by a tiny crack in the concept of practices providing total care for their patients.

At about this time, the three-year vocational training schemes for general practice were developing in different parts of the country, and Christopher became one of the first two trainers in the town. From a practice's point of view, the scheme provided intellectual stimulation and another pair of hands. It also brought a useful stream of potential partners.

Despite the advances already mentioned, the workload was getting heavier and the therapeutic opportunities increasing; the practice needed an additional partner. I was on the training scheme at the time, and in 1974 we agreed that I should join them on completion of my training the following year.

Jim stayed on a few years before retiring. He was stone deaf in one ear and possibly not a lot better in the other. Consequently, he always found meetings trying. He would sit quietly at partnership meetings, probably largely disengaged – you could never be sure. Then, at a time Jim considered reasonable he, as senior partner, would suddenly stand up and declare the meeting over, sometimes with someone else in mid-sentence!

Nonetheless, in the early 1970s, he was chair of the local medical committee, the professional body representing local GPs. He retired in 1980, a much loved and deeply respected GP. His successor was Allan Leroy, another doctor in the training scheme who, like me a few years earlier, had come to us for his final year.

And so, we were four, Drs Elliott-Binns, Woolmore, Willis, and Leroy, and we remained that way for many years. It was to be the last partnership of full-timers in a history dating back nearly one and a half centuries. Of course, the practice would continue. It would evolve and improve immeasurably regarding its clinical abilities, its premises, organisation, staff, and technology. But the previous singular unity of purpose would, for better and for worse, be gone for good.

TRAINING TO BE A GP

My hope for this chapter is that it gives some flavour of daily life as a junior doctor in the early 1970s.

***

Every teaching hospital has its traditions and celebrities, and at the Middlesex in 1974 Arthur was one such, though he would only claim to be a minor one.[19] He kept himself to himself, always to be found hanging around in the Fracture Clinic, near Casualty. He was usually in the lockers, those narrow, green metal cabinets with clanging doors so often found in the changing rooms of sports clubs. Occasionally, he put in an appearance, but usually he stayed quietly in his home, for Arthur was a skeleton.

Within our first days at medical school, we had to buy half a skeleton (for some reason from Dillons bookshop in Gower Street); it was a rite of passage. Only one half for three reasons. First, it saved money. Half price, you might say. Second, presumably, it made the available bodies go further, though I have not studied the supply chain in depth. And third, you only needed one of each bone. Once you have seen one fibula, you have seen them all.

What we bought with pride in those first few days was just a brown cardboard box full of jumbled bones, the longest a femur – which defined the length of the box. The *pièce de résistance* was a complete skull that laid on the top of the pile. I accept that, on the face of it, this seems to contradict my second advantage of half-skeletons. Perhaps, somewhere there is a market for headless half-skeletons.

---

[19] The Middlesex has gone now – demolished – with the proceeds absorbed into the new, vast, green-glazed University College Hospital on the Euston Road. Only the Grade II listed 1929 chapel remains, standing defiantly in the middle of developers' tower blocks.

Arthur looked with disdain on his hemi-cousins. He was the real McCoy,[20] the Rolls-Royce Silver Ghost of skeletons. Not only was he complete but, crucially, he had that extra something, that extra panache. Arthur was articulated, his bones wired together, so he dangled, Halloween-style, from a hook screwed into the top of his skull.

I mention Arthur here because he and I were to share what, for me at least, was an unforgettable experience.

HOW NOT TO GET FROM A TO B WITHOUT CAUSING C

My first job was as one of the two orthopaedic house surgeons at the Middlesex Hospital in central London. I was interested in orthopaedics as a career, in part reflecting my long-held interest in constructing things.

One morning, my fellow houseman James and I were asked to take Arthur to the hospital's Courtauld lecture theatre for a lunchtime demonstration. It was our job because the Fracture Clinic was in our domain, and that is where Arthur lived.

What at first sight seemed a simple task became more complicated as we confronted Arthur, who was grinning at us from inside his green, metal home. The Middlesex, constructed in the early 1930s, was H-shaped and six red-brick storeys high, its two wings joined by a central crosspiece. The lecture theatre was on the third-floor crosspiece, at the centre of the hospital, while the Fracture Clinic was on the ground floor of the west wing. So, our route would inevitably take us along the hospital's bustling corridors, teeming with early morning staff and patients.

Worse, on that morning our west wing lifts were out of order.

---

[20] The real thing; the genuine article. The expression first appears as the real Mackay, with real possibly being a corruption of the name of the Reay branch of the Scottish Mackay family.

Accordingly, we had no choice but to traverse the full width of the hospital on the ground floor, including crossing the back of the large and impressive entrance hall, where both visitors and new admissions first reported. We would then arrive at the east wing lifts. From there it would be easy – assuming no patients were in the lift – for once on the third floor we could come back along the crosspiece corridor to the lecture theatre. That was the plan.

The more we thought about it, the more complicated it all became. We could hardly walk through the hospital carrying a skeleton dangling from a metal drip stand, particularly if we had to cross the main entrance hall where new patients sat in rows, waiting for direction to their appropriate ward and without the need of seeing a skeleton walking past them. We concluded it would be more discreet to put Arthur on a hospital trolley for the journey, covering him with a sheet.

But then we thought again. Patients on trolleys are a commonplace in any hospital, but if the only visible part is the head of a skeleton, this could alarm at least some of those we passed. We decided to pull the sheet right over Arthur, covering him completely.

But that would not do either. The world over, the only patients on trolleys with their heads concealed in this way, both in films and reality, are dead ones; or as John Cleese might say, ex-patients.[21] Arthur was certainly that, but surely we could not trundle an apparent corpse along hospital corridors while patients politely stood aside to let us pass?

Despite all, this seemed to be the best option. We laid Arthur on a casualty trolley, covering him with a freshly laundered, white hospital sheet, and set off. James was at the front, and I manned the back, both in our white coats and Arthur well covered. We went down the west

---

[21] One of several euphemisms for death ("is no more", "has ceased to be", "bereft of life, it rests in peace", and "this is an ex-parrot") used in the celebrated and very funny Monty Python's *Dead Parrot* sketch.

wing corridor and around the right-hand corner towards the main entrance hall. All was going well.

But then, I regret to say, I was overcome by my innate sense of the comically absurd. With one of those inappropriate emotional responses that can afflict any of us at just the wrong moment, I began to smile. And then to grin. It must have been the thought of Arthur's face beneath the sheet and the farcical nature of the occasion.

Now, a body covered from head to toe with a white sheet being pushed through a busy hospital on a trolley in the middle of the morning is bad enough, but when one of the "porters" in attendance is grinning inanely from ear to ear, the scene is brushed with the macabre. We had to do something.

"Speed up, James," I hissed in alarm. We sped up.

Unfortunately, this made matters worse. We must have presented an unfortunate picture, hurrying a trolley along the corridor, transporting what appeared to be a deceased patient, at a speed that would make any funeral director shake their head in dismay. Worse still, one of the two attendants was now actually laughing.

But – true to farce – things were to deteriorate further when we arrived at the back of the front hall, complete with its rows of anxious patients awaiting admission. The hospital's large entrance doors were now to our right and our path to the east wing straight ahead. Now, that mischievous joker serendipity spotted an opportunity and joined in the fun. Someone opened the front doors wide, admitting a wintry blast of air.

Due to a combination of the gust of wind and the speed of the trolley, the leading edge of the sheet lifted. At first, it was just a little, and then – like a spinnaker filled with wind – it began to balloon and rise, exposing part of Arthur to anyone who happened to be watching. Our only option was to increase speed still further, grabbing at the sheet to hold it down, and we departed the scene as quickly as possible.

I hoped we had vanished into the east wing and the relative solitude of the bank of lifts before people realised what was going on; perhaps they were distracted by the opening doors and the cold draught. Once out of sight, we adjusted Arthur's covering, entered a lift, which was indeed empty, closed the doors and completed our journey to the lecture theatre, all without further mishap.

***

In many ways, that orthopaedic job was the happiest in my short career as a junior hospital doctor. I was working with two exceptional consultants who would remain unknowing influences throughout my career. Philip "Pip" Newman was the elder statesman, a gentle bear of a man, veteran of Second World War medicine, the man chosen to repair Churchill's fractured femur, an expert in spinal disorders and the Secretary of the British Orthopaedic Association. Rodney Sweetnam was the young pretender, the youngest consultant to have been appointed to the Middlesex and who was later to become the knighted President of the Royal College of Surgeons. To work with those two was hugely exciting for a newly minted doctor. They knew I was interested in orthopaedics and gave me every opportunity to develop that interest both on the wards and the operating theatre, and offered their personal support in guiding my future career.

It was against that heady backdrop that I realised orthopaedics was not for me. Despite being an exciting, constructive clinical discipline, it was too specialised and too constrained for what I wanted. And since then, like all specialities, it has become even more so, and ever more focused on technical procedures. That is fine if you have a passion for a career in a narrowing aspect of a particular discipline. I have great respect for specialists and their expertise. But it was not for me.

I wanted a career that embraced the whole panoply of medicine, one that took a holistic approach to the patient, and allowed me autonomy to develop my work and its environment in ways a small group of colleagues and I wanted. That was a million miles from hospital medicine but described general practice very well.

For many doctors, it was the real thing. It spans medicine, from toes and tumours to lungs and livers, from helping individuals not only to stay alive but to live, and it deals with the broad subtleties of the mind. As I said earlier, it is now the NHS in microcosm, covering prevention, acute care, and chronic disease management, and spanning the years from before birth to just after death.[22] And at that time, we could develop our practices almost entirely as we felt best, developing our buildings, information systems, and personnel. No other branch of medicine offered the freedom to flex your creativity across such a broad field.

I was sorry to leave the orthopaedic department, with its class-leading standards, closely knit team, and the happy ability to lunch each day off the limitless chocolates brought in as presents for the nurses. Black Magic were my favourites, but Dairy Milk came in a close second.

***

In the early 1970s, accommodation for junior doctors working at the Middlesex was in the residential wing of the main building. Deductions for board and lodging wiped out most of our salary, but in any case, there was not much time to go out and spend it. We were all working throughout the day and on call alternate nights and weekends. But we were lucky. The cardiothoracic house surgeon had a particularly challenging time. There was only one of him, and so he

---

[22] Legally and contractually, a person ceases to be your patient at the moment of death, but there are still niceties to be undertaken, and in any case, the deceased's family are likely to be patients as well, and they will have needs of their own. At the other end of life, there is a professional responsibility to the mother's unborn baby, though you cannot register a child with an NHS GP until after birth.

was on duty continuously for the whole six months, even sleeping every night on the ward to be available as quickly as possible. He seldom left the hospital, a traditional highlight being one evening off in the entire six months as a favour from the registrar. After a few months, you could spot the holder of that job by his prison pallor. Typical of 1970s thinking, the hospital's bigwigs deemed the post unsuitable for fragile females, while presumably being perfectly acceptable for the hardier sex.

A pair of married doctors was something of a novelty for the residency's staff. We arrived to find we had two rooms, which was very nice, except mine was on the third floor and Eunice's on the fifth. We told them that we thought we would manage with just the one.

"Very well," the rather Edwardian housekeeper said. "We will bring the second bed down to the third-floor room."

Her expression did flicker for a moment when I said we would not require the second bed either, in part because we needed room for the workbench. I have no idea what she thought its purpose to be.

Our single room made an adequately cosy home. It was a bit cramped, but we ate our meals in the junior staff dining room downstairs and were busy on the wards all day. On call alternate nights, either one of us could be up to visit the wards; occasionally both at the same time. Our room was a bit of a transit camp, though I managed to build a pair of large loudspeakers when not at work. These were to replace Tom and Jerry, which I had abandoned in the basement of Astor College when we left. The maintenance technicians allowed me to use the hospital's workshops for a particularly tricky bit of routing, and the curator of instruments drooled over my grandmother's carving tools. His primary job was to maintain and sharpen the instruments used for operations. (Disposable scalpels were by now available, but the older styles preferred by some surgeons required sharpening by hand.) The carving chisels were made from Sheffield steel at a time when that was the best. He took them away, returning them in absolutely magnificent condition, cleaned and scalpel sharp! I still use them.

***

Domestic life improved when we moved on from the Middlesex, to work as junior doctors at Salisbury Royal Infirmary.[23] The hospital was situated centrally in the city, and we lived with four other junior doctors in a wonderful old, ivy-covered house in the grounds, where, being married, we were allocated a small flat. We were two of the three medical house physicians and so on duty much of the time, but it was another happy, compact, and largely self-sufficient medical community. There was the regional hospital in Southampton, but for most cases, Salisbury managed everything that came its way.

Of course, there were exceptions to that self-contained tradition. We needed the services of the neurosurgical department at Southampton for one. The unfortunate patient had been working on a building site before the law required hard hats. (He may have been a statistic that helped promote that law, but not even a glass fibre hat would have helped on this occasion.)

He was standing under some scaffolding when, from high above, one of his workmates accidentally dropped a steel reinforcing rod, one of those used to strengthen concrete. The thin javelin fell several floors and went straight through the poor man's head. A ghoulish problem confronted the ambulance crew. The long bar sticking through his head meant he could not fit through the door of the ambulance, so the fire brigade was summoned, and they carefully cut off each end before gently loading him into the vehicle.

---

[23] Sadly, it was demolished some years later when all services transferred to Odstock Road a few miles away. I am sure that made good economic sense to someone.

Of course, he was lucky not to have been killed at once; some head injuries are like that.[24] On arrival at our hospital, he was still alive but unconscious and needed urgent transfer to a neurosurgical unit. Outside Casualty, the medical registrar on duty took charge and, no doubt with relief, immediately redirected the ambulance 25 miles to Southampton. He then phoned the neurosurgeons to say the man was on his way.

The young admitting doctor in Southampton agreed completely.

"OK. Just give me the details. What's the patient's name?"

"I'm afraid I've no idea," said the registrar, still shaken by the event.

"Well, I really should have his name. What's his date of birth?"

"I'm afraid I don't know that either."

"I must have these details. We get a large number of admissions. I have to be able to tell which is which."

"Well, I tell you what," said the rather more experienced registrar. "If you get more than one patient in the next hour with a reinforcing rod stuck through his head, then phone me back, and I'll try to describe the one coming from Salisbury." He rang off.

Young admitting doctors all too often asked silly questions, wherever they worked. I remember doing it and probably more than most, though this case taught me to try to avoid it. It reflects the pedantry of professional immaturity; not knowing yet when to bend the rules, when to break free and trust the intangibles of common sense. Other occupations also have their jobsworths; they are invariably annoying.

---

[24] Perhaps the most famous case was the American railroad worker Phineas P Gage. In 1848, he was using a tamping rod weighing about 12 lb to compress explosive powder. Unfortunately, a spark caused an explosion, and the rod shot vertically through his head to land about 30 yards away. Phineas survived but suffered an altered personality. Interest in his case precipitated the development of surgical lobotomy for some psychiatric conditions.

Even in Salisbury, I managed to fit in some woodwork. If I was not working on Sunday afternoons, I was allowed to use the hospital's carpentry workshop. It provided a couple of hours of complete change and relaxation, working at the bench while listening to Sam Costa on the transistor radio there. I made a dressing table mirror out of Honduras mahogany – a copy of one by Gordon Russell I had seen photographed in a book. It is still in our bedroom over 40 years later.

Some evenings, I sat in with local GPs to see their work. It is an indictment of six years of medical training that this was my first experience of general practice. That would be true of almost every doctor at that stage, yet half of them were to become GPs.

***

No sooner had you started a six-month hospital house job, than it was time to plan the next one. After Salisbury, I had completed my compulsory preregistration year of surgery and medicine. It was time to focus on general practice.

Training programmes had just emerged. Previously, there had been informal, commonly exploitative opportunities of one sort or another for young GPs, but emerging now were the structured vocational training programmes that followed the pioneering work of Dr George Swift in the Wessex Region during the 1960s and reports from the College of GPs (CGP).[25] At the end of a three-year rotation course, provided everything had gone well, you could apply for a partnership as someone who had been signed off as a competent GP.

They were still a novelty, and voluntary. In 1971, there were only 11 available in the whole country, offering a total of about 60 places a year. In contrast, after 1982 every doctor wishing to enter general practice had to undertake such training. By 2010, there were courses

---

[25] College of General Practitioners (1965). *Reports from General Practice. I. Special Vocational Training for General Practice.* London, Council of the College of General Practitioners.

everywhere and over 3000 places available. They all start after the compulsory first year of hospital work in medicine and surgery. Typically, they involve two more years of hospital work, rotating through a series of relevant specialities such as children's medicine, gynaecology, and obstetrics, followed by a year in a training practice.

Most of those to which I wrote in 1971 were already full, but for several reasons, the one at Northampton General Hospital caught my eye. It had better facilities than the others, a brand-new postgraduate centre, and uniquely (at that time) it split the 36 months equally between training practices and hospital. Better again, it boasted a higher pay scale. The course was set up by the excellent postgraduate clinical tutor, Dr Ted Sever, who told us he felt Eunice could get work in the hospital as well, as indeed she did.

The course turned out to be a good choice. The first year involved six months of obstetrics and gynaecology followed by six months of paediatrics. Both are essential to general practice. Children make good patients and in various ways, paediatrics is general medicine in miniature. It also taught you to acquire new skills and be confident in their use. For example, putting intravenous infusions into tiny, very ill babies at 3:00 a.m. when you have just woken up can be a severe challenge for the most skilled clinician. You become justly proud of acquiring such skills. Later, you are amazed at how quickly they fade with disuse.

The beginning of my second year, in 1972, took me to a rural practice in Moulton, a stone village just north of Northampton, where John Campling was my first GP trainer. The practice had a new building and dispensary; the single storey design was very typical of rather harsh, early 1970s architecture. There were two partners, pleasant staff, a beautiful rural practice area, and an air of caring competence that befitted its excellent reputation. Even the weather was kind. It was incredibly exciting.

My first day was memorable, not just because of the excitement, but because things nearly went very wrong indeed. As usual, after morning surgery the partners shared out the list of requests for home visits. "Andrew, have you ever seen a case of measles?"

I had not. (Incidentally, this in itself was remarkable, especially since I had just finished six winter months of paediatrics. It reflected well on the NHS immunisation programme, a vital public health programme since buffeted by episodes of mischievous, misinforming media speculation.)

"There is a case here you can go and see, and it's in one of the outlying villages so you'll get a chance to drive around the practice area and get to know it."

I set off, full of the joys of spring, briefed on the diagnosis and management of measles, roaring along the narrow, empty country roads in my new Triumph Spitfire, a prize of employment. After I found the cottage, the patient's mother showed me into the living room where a boy was lying on the sofa. He looked very ill indeed.

Here my guardian angel smiled again. As I had said to my trainers, I had never seen a measles rash before that consultation, and I still had not afterwards. But by remarkable good fortune, during my paediatrics job, I had seen the rash of meningococcal septicaemia. There had been a mini outbreak, and I had dealt with five cases in the hospital – every one, incidentally, diagnosed correctly by the patient's GP.

Back in the cottage, the diagnosis was made, an antibiotic injection given, hospital alerted, emergency ambulance called, and the boy loaded on board.

A rather shaken, second year GP trainee drove slowly back to the practice. "Avoid preconceptions" is a useful rule in medicine, as it is elsewhere, though a tough one to follow. I shall refer to it again.

No one was at fault here, and no one was exceptionally smart. We were all lucky; that is all. The mother had seen a rash and assumed it was measles, so she phoned the practice and told the receptionist. The reason given on the visiting list we studied over coffee only said the boy had measles. We had to visit, not only to assess the patient but also to confirm the diagnosis – though usually not dangerous, measles is a notifiable disease.

There was much less publicity about meningococcal meningitis then than there is now, and it was pure chance that the young doctor who visited happened to have seen several cases only weeks before. It could so easily have been different. A senior GP would probably have recognised the rash, as demonstrated by the five cases I saw in the hospital, but the doctor who entered the house that day did so on his first day in general practice, preprogrammed to see his first case of measles, and to learn the appearance of the rash. Fortune smiled on us all. How different might the outcome have been? And how would it have read in the press? "Boy dies when training GP mistakes killer meningitis for measles."

The patient received prompt treatment at the hospital and returned home after a couple of weeks.

That is the reality of medicine, and particularly general practice. No matter how good the training, how good the support, nor how experienced we are, some set of circumstances will always come along influenced by fortune. Some of those will include the potential for far-reaching consequences.

***

After the village practice at Moulton, there were six months rotating around appropriate hospital outpatient clinics, and looking after the rheumatology ward where I could pursue my persisting, partial interest in orthopaedic medicine.

The final year was with another trainer, Christopher Elliott-Binns. His practice was the one in Billing Road where I had undertaken that first locum session two years earlier. Here, for the first time, I had my own consulting room, and I was very proud of it. Yes, it was in the basement at the back of the house, and yes, it was underground and needed the lights on all the time. But there was a window looking out to a sort of gully behind the house and, if you looked up at an acute angle, you could see the sky. There was a gas fire for cold days and, ready for my arrival, the practice had obtained a date stamp with my name on it. Few things could make you feel more at home than for your name to be on the consulting room door the morning you arrived, and for there to be a personalised date stamp on the desk.

Certainly, the back wall of the room was damp, and not infrequently stained with patches of black mould, but little in life is perfect, and the room was mine. At one stage I sprayed the mould with a sample canister of clotrimazole antifungal medication given to me by a pharmaceutical company rep. Now you can buy it over the counter, but do not bother trying it on a black mould; my experiment was a resounding failure. Unlike the athlete's foot which was the intended target for the spray, the mould on the wall did not seem to mind my treatment one bit. The only change was that now the black patches were shiny, covered by a clear film, and even more apparent than before.

It was all because of a faulty downpipe outside the back door of the consulting room, from which steps led up to the back garden. There was always the threat that the downpipe would give up completely when faced with torrential rains, and indeed that is what happened. One wintry afternoon I was in the middle of a consultation, the gas fire hissing hypnotically in the background and the rain pouring down outside when I realised I was losing my patient's attention. Behind me, water was coming underneath the door from the garden and – not so slowly – edging under my chair, creeping across the carpet towards him.

He was a pragmatic sort of man and once he had pointed out the unwelcome ingress we used towels to block up the gap under the door, mopped the floor with paper from the examination couch, and resumed our consultation, the room gently suffused by a smell of wet carpet drying before the fire. That sort of spontaneous interlude has a certain charm but does not seem to happen as much now.

The few of us who were on the training scheme wanted to develop it. We already had a day release course in Aylesbury every month, organised by the Oxford Region's postgraduate office, but though a pleasant day off it did not hit the spot. We wanted to arrange our own local and weekly half-day release for training. Our Northampton course organiser was supportive and, despite initial incredulity from the hospital consultants, we got our half-day off a week for training – a novelty at that time for junior doctors. Time set aside for learning how to do your job was not something that happened in hospital medicine. But crucially, we GP trainees were the first junior grade hospital doctors not to be beholden to our consultants for career advancement. Such liberty allowed us an arrogant determination to ensure our training scheme met our needs. It must have been a difficult pill for the consultants to swallow, but it taught me the power of independent GPs who wanted change. It was a lesson I would remember 20 years later.

The training half-day was a great success, and I think continues to this day. There were other ways we all tried to push the Northampton training scheme forward. We wanted to try video recording our consultations, and reviewing them afterwards. All this must sound very introspective and self-righteous, but in mitigation, two things are worth pointing out. Vocational training at that time was very new and entirely voluntary. We did not have to do it to become a GP principal, as became the case a few years later. And that leads to the second point, that by delaying our appointments to partnerships by two years we were taking a not insignificant financial hit. Junior doctors' pay scales did not equate to those of GP principals. In effect, we were paying to go on the course, so it had to be worth our while. Currently, universities will be only too familiar with such attitudes from their fee-paying students.

Video recording consultations is commonplace now, but it certainly was not then. In fact, we got the idea from a patient describing the process in his industrial training. A pharmaceutical company agreed to lend us some video equipment, and we created a set of personalities and scenarios for John Campling's amateur dramatic group to role-play as patients.

Afterwards, everyone gathered around for the viewings, with a couple of our trainers acting as tutors, analysts, counsellors, and riot police. The most valuable lesson was to hear what the actors thought. There is no reason to believe that we were the very first to do this, but we were among the first, and it was fun, some years later, to see the technique introduced into GP vocational training schemes as the latest thing in medical education!

And therein lies another observation. At that time, everything was so new that we could shape our course in ways we felt would best help us. Neither we nor the course had to conform to the ideas of someone else. It was new, exciting, and free-spirited, and our trainers supported us in our efforts to innovate in ways we, the users, thought best. Organisations are all the better for that.

And so, my vocational training drew to a happy close. I was what both the Royal College of GPs (RCGP) and the NHS now refer to – at first glance oxymoronically – as a specialist generalist, and I accepted the invitation to stay on as a partner at the Billing Road surgery.

DOES ANYONE KNOW WHAT WE ARE TRYING TO DO?

"What exactly are we trying to do? How are we going to do it, and how are we going to do it better?"

These were just the sort of questions the new brand of GP trainees in the early 1970s asked their training practices. Perhaps it reflected a liberal 1960s education; perhaps trainees had time to entertain such whimsical thoughts, displaying a naïve, coltish inquisitiveness. But they were sensible questions. Surely, we needed to know what we were trying to do. Nothing at medical school, nor in our careers to date had touched on such issues.

Surprisingly, few precise answers were forthcoming. After all, it was explained, a GP simply did what a GP did. That our trainers could not define their job in objective terms led to a momentary wonder as to how they hoped to train others to do it.

Although there were notable exceptions, at that time few GPs took a calculated interest in managing the service provision of their practices.[26] In the 1970s, the profession – even at its highest levels – either minimised or disregarded the significance of management. During my three years in a vocational training scheme, no time at all was given to studying management techniques that could be used later in our practices. Remember that GPs are independent, self-employed doctors who contract their services to the NHS. They are not employees, like hospital doctors; they run businesses (though, coyly, in my day they hated to think of their practices as such). It would seem reasonable for their trainees to assume they had an interest in what they were trying to do, how they were doing it, and with what

---

[26] Even now, management has an unfortunate stigma in the eyes of many, but it is a necessity for getting anything done.

results. But we were wrong. There was little interest in the objective analysis of what practices did.

Indeed, as I recall, the national arrangements for funding postgraduate education expressly excluded subjects concerned with organisational management. They were not appropriate; we were not allowed to do those! Enlightened local organisers occasionally included them, but only hidden as a discrete part of a broader, clinical subject.

If the office for postgraduate education at Oxford Regional Health Authority (RHA) considered a session to be on management rather than a clinical topic, then – astonishingly – that session would not be authorised. A rare medical condition that, in all probability, we would never see was perfectly acceptable, but the structured management of a practice's 200 patients with diabetes was not. We trainees rightly thought this madness.

Let me be clear. I am not thinking of management regarding making money and accounting. We were not trainee hedge funders. I am talking about organisational management subjects, such as how to provide a programme of preventive medicine for our patients, or how to survey them to see how they felt we could improve the services offered. But our elders and betters, people who would consider it stupid not to take a map on a long walk in the country to plan their route and check on progress, here felt such assessment activities were inappropriate for the young professionals they were training.

Of course, we needed to learn about clinical care in general practice, for it differed from hospital medicine both in its case mix and management. But what we knew nothing about, nothing at all, was how to run a practice. We knew nothing about how to look after the holistic care of a registered list of several thousand patients – a cornerstone of general practice yet something beyond our previous hospital experience. We knew nothing about how to organise staff, decide objectives for the practice, and then assess results against them.

About these issues, we were taught nothing unless we arranged the training ourselves.[27,28]

There was a clear reason. Throughout the country, with a few notable exceptions, the trainers did not know either. Of even greater significance was that, to come perilously close to quoting Donald Rumsfeld, they did not know that they did not know.

The trainers were not alone in having difficulty describing the role of a GP; it was proving surprisingly difficult for everyone. Even the National Health Service Act 1997 threw in the towel, describing the duty of GPs as "to render to their patients all necessary and appropriate medical services of the type usually provided by general practitioners."

Such a circuitous definition did not help very much. It reflected the earlier Bolam principle used by the courts as one part of the determination of professional negligence.[29] No wonder there was variability in the standards and services offered by several thousand individual practices. Each was free to follow its own priorities, methods, and standards, provided that it did roughly what most others did. And in any case, who was to know what most other GPs did? There were few if any relevant measures.

The wonder is not that GPs were different, but that they were so similar. It is remarkable that even in the early 1970s very few had ever formally studied another doctor doing the same job, even for a few days. It would not be until the mid-1990s that over half had done so.

Before the advent of training schemes in the late 1960s, it was as if each GP inhabited his own Darwinian Galapagos island. They were

---

[27] Confusingly the word "management" has always been used in medicine for the clinical care of individuals, as in "the management of her pneumonia", but until the 1970s clinicians shunned it for organisational matters on a larger scale.
[28] Willis A (1984). The need for management training in the postgraduate education of general practitioners. *J R Coll Gen Pract*, 34(259): 116–117.
[29] The Bolam principle states that "if a doctor reaches the standard of a responsible body of medical opinion, he is not negligent."

isolated both professionally and socially, and though their methods evolved in adaptation to their particular environments, overall they worked along remarkably similar lines. They might have different beaks, but they were still finches.

One explanation is that the essence of the job in the 1950s was reactive, and its organisation quite straightforward. Anyone wanting a medical opinion would go to the family doctor, or ask for a home visit. The doctor's task was to identify the problem and do what was possible to alleviate symptoms, or even cure their cause, preferably without causing too much harm in the process. Some did it well, and some did it badly. Sometimes it was straightforward, at other times complex. But in essence that was the task; it was a reactive one they all shared.

THE DAWN OF OPPORTUNITY

But in the 1970s things became more complicated, with opportunities appearing that could expand the range of services provided. First, these involved the management of ongoing conditions, such as diabetes and heart disease. Second, it became possible to provide a broad range of preventive services right across Shakespeare's seven ages of man, though I must say little was done for his whining schoolboy.

This point was critical. These new services were practice-led and optional. The doctors decided whether or not to offer a service; they invited patients, and the patients chose whether or not to respond. If previously the medical intervention had been triggered by the patient, these new ones were by invitation. This ball game was a new one, and the meandering crack in the ice that had always divided the standards of practices now opened into a crevasse.

For many GPs, these new ideas involved an irrational, uneconomic use of their time and money. Of course, you could do them – you were autonomous and self-employed – but you did them in your own time and at your own expense.

Inevitably, practices took different views as to whether they should set up such systems. Some tried, using paper registers and a lot of hard work, but progress was limited. Most practices, arguably with sense on their side, did not even try. When eventually real progress was made, it came in the 1980s, with financial help for employing additional staff, but more than anything else because of the availability of computers. Even then, at first only innovative practices took up the silicon baton and ran with it.

***

At last, a clear definition of the work of a GP appeared in 1972 when the RCGP published *The Future General Practitioner*. The book did not have the broad-based impact that it deserved. It contained a careful description of a GP's work that was taken up and amended two years later by the second European Conference on the Teaching of General Practice.

As time has passed, the definition has been refined into wordy statements that embrace cultural and societal change, their clumsy complexity indicative of their derivation within large committees. The first third of one produced by the European Region of the World Organization of Family Doctors (WONCA)[30] is reproduced here, even if its first sentence is gratingly ugly:

> *General practitioners/family doctors are specialist physicians trained in the principles of the discipline. They are personal doctors, primarily responsible for the provision of comprehensive and continuing care to every individual seeking medical care irrespective of age, sex and illness. They care for*

---

[30] WONCA is the unusual, yet convenient acronym comprising the first five initials of the World Organization of National Colleges, Academies and Academic Associations of General Practitioners/Family Physicians.

individuals in the context of their family, their community, and their culture, always respecting the autonomy of their patients.[31]

Here we should pause to consider that last sentence, for general practice is concerned with far more than treating acute conditions presented by an individual. Of course, it involves the individual, but it also deals with groups of people, that is to say, populations. A real understanding of general practice, and indeed of the NHS, requires us to appreciate the significance of the concentric populations that are so difficult to describe. But try I must, for it is a central theme to much of this book.

CONCENTRIC POPULATIONS

Any individual patient is at the centre of a series of ever larger populations, like the rings in a pool of water caused by a dropped pebble, its effects spreading further and further from the centre with progressively diminishing force. The patient – you or me – is the pebble, the immediate focus that drops into the consulting room, but the outer rings have significance too.

The one nearest the centre is the patient's family or closest group. Very few people have no inner group at all. Outside that lies the practice's list of several thousand patients, and beyond that the local community, then the town and on to the region and country. Picture an enormous plate balanced on a pin positioned below its centre. Then imagine people distributed evenly around the plate, each standing on its edge. If we move the plate below any one of the individuals, then to a greater or lesser extent we move each of the others. What we do to one influences all the others. It is not possible to do otherwise and

---

[31] WONCA Europe (2011). *The European Definition of General Practice/Family Medicine*. [online] Available from: http://tinyurl.com/pjzfcjz (accessed 9 January 2017).

the plate remains on the pin. Too big a movement under one person and the whole thing collapses.

We cannot treat one individual without regard for others; neither can we, as patients, expect to be treated without such regard. For some that is a harsh truth, even an unacceptable one to be denied, but it applies throughout medicine, whether in the NHS or, albeit to a lesser extent, within private care.

To illustrate the point, we can consider an example. A patient is consulting a doctor – let us say privately to emphasise the commonality of the issue. During the discussion, it transpires that the patient's initially simple presentation has multiple ramifications. Together, these would take an hour or so, but her appointment is only for 30 minutes. Now the doctor has a problem. They may elect to slightly overrun to deal with as much as possible, and then arrange to address the remaining issues at another time. The hour the patient requires is simply not available because other patients are waiting. They also have appointments, and their problems may be of equal or even greater clinical importance.[32]

So here, as always, the doctor addresses the requirements of the individual within the context of a larger population. In the example, that larger population is all the patients due to be seen in the consulting session.

In other circumstances, the relevant populations may be much larger. The collective needs of a GP's registered list of several thousand patients must be considered in the context of an even larger one – the population of the community or town. GPs may feel several of their patients are in particular need of urgent hospital treatment. However, the hospital has a broader catchment population than just their practice, and it may be that there are other patients, from other practices, who are even more deserving of priority access. Those with

---

[32] That is the theory. However, throughout my career, I was appalling at keeping to time, as any of my patients would attest.

the greater need should go first. It is the lifeboat principle: the weaker and most in need go first. In medicine, equity should trump selfishness and equality. We may be next in the Accident and Emergency (A & E) queue with our cut finger, but the man rushed in with a heart attack jumps in front of us, and few would think that wrong.[33]

I repeat, lest there still be doubt: this principle is not peculiar to the NHS. A private patient may feel their own needs are of supreme priority, but if their specialist has others with greater clinical needs, then professional ethics decree that these should be dealt with first, no matter how indignant a patient may become. Unless you have your own, full-time personal doctor – and very few people in the world do – this applies in any system and anywhere.

Clinicians often fudge the principle. "My only duty is to the patient in front of me" is a commendable professional mantra, but it is wrong, or at best simplistic. The preceding paragraphs illustrate that taken literally, it cannot be so. A more accurate statement would be that a clinician's responsibility to the patient in front of them is to do the very best they can, given the resources available to them. That distinction is not petty pedantry: it is a fundamental principle that underpins healthcare.

So, the word "population" refers at different times to different groups of people. In the first example, it means the group of patients with appointments for that particular consulting session. In the second, it refers to all the patients on a surgeon's waiting list in the local hospital. Those patients should be managed equitably, according to their relative need compared to the other patients who are also waiting. That relative need may change again should they be referred to a regional centre, with its even larger catchment population. And it may change in the blink of an eye, as anyone knows who has had an

---

[33] People are always "rushed" to hospital, no matter what is wrong with them. Journalists seldom avoid that verb!

operation cancelled at the last moment because of a new, emergency admission that requires urgent surgery.

Later we shall see how ignoring this fundamental of medical practice created a fatal fault line in a major government health policy.

ANSWERING THE QUESTIONS

By the later 1970s, our practice was providing a planned service on three broad fronts: acute care, preventive care, and chronic disease management. This was a very different game to the reactive service the practice had provided only a few years previously.

The RCGP's overall aim, described at length in 1972, was too nebulous for the needs of many practices. We preferred to construct our own succinct and pragmatic description:

> *To provide high-quality acute care to all who seek it, and preventive care and chronic disease management to those registered with the practice.*[34]

We created the organisational structure for achieving our aim through developing the right buildings, personnel, systems, and management, and we created a conceptual framework for providing services to appropriate cohorts of patients defined by age and sex for preventive purposes, or by diagnostic group for chronic disease management. In 1980, we produced our first annual report, with measured outcomes set against specific objectives for different elements of the practice, and new targets were then established for the following year.

With such an organisation in place, practices such as ours could begin to answer those original questions. What exactly are we trying to do? How are we getting on? How are we going to do it better?

---

[34] The national contract for GPs required us to provide immediately necessary care to anyone who requested it, whether registered with the practice or not. It made no mention of prevention or chronic disease management.

PART TWO

A BRIEF HISTORY OF NHS GENERAL PRACTICE

We all have views about the NHS, ranging from love to loathing, but how much do we actually know about it? Where did it come from, and how has it developed? On the basis of what knowledge do we form our opinions?

Before we can comment about anything with any authority, we need an adequate amount of background knowledge, yet most of us feel free to express opinions about the NHS – an organisation costing over £110 billion a year – based on our singular experience, or that of friends, family, and newspaper editors.

Part Two makes no pretence to being an exhaustive history of the NHS, but at least it provides a sketch, a summary, of the key features from which modern general practice evolved.

THE EARLY DAYS OF THE NHS

Despite frequent criticism, the NHS is the part of our society that the British most cherish. Politically, the NHS is not so much a hot potato as a nuclear trigger. In 1992, Nigel Lawson referred to it as "the closest thing the English have to a national religion."[35] In 2010, and again in 2014, it received higher levels of public satisfaction than ever before, much to the delight of politicians trying to weather the storms of criticism for their spending cuts. Screams of real anger are inevitable against anyone – of any political persuasion – who is thought to be threatening the fundamental principles of the NHS.

We think of the NHS much as parents may view their teenage offspring. Perhaps we do not know as much about them as we should; perhaps we do not have much control over them. But they are ours; they are family. We can criticise them as much as we like, but we love them dearly, and God help anyone else who says a bad word about them.

For most UK citizens, the same applies to the NHS. We may criticise it ourselves, but will defend it if others do so. We laugh at Americans who criticise it from their position of self-centred dogma and ignorance, and we despair at the arrogance of private hospitals that claim superiority while relying on the NHS to provide intensive care beds when they need them. In general, despite its shortcomings, the NHS is perceived as simply a good thing. It is a wholesome contrast to the failings of our society: of egocentric bankers and their bulging bonuses; of inexplicable road rage; of child abuse; phone hacking scandals; the infuriatingly elusive language of politicians; and of wars of questionable purpose and morality.

That said, for some, the NHS is an appalling waste of money. To

---

[35] Lawson N (1992). *The View from No.11: Memoirs of a Tory Radical.* London, Bantam Press, p. 613.

them, it is inefficient and bureaucratic, irrefutably inferior to services provided by the private sector, and a remnant of old socialist ideologies. They argue for their share of the money spent on the NHS and that they will then make better use of it. Such a case is appealing to the young and healthy, even as it completely misses the point of risk sharing across a population. Attitudes can change when these critics develop a long-term illness of their own, such as renal failure or rheumatoid arthritis. Suddenly, health insurance can be found wanting, even for those who started the policy before the condition's onset. Conversely, others argue that it can fail some people because of the severe nature of their condition. In this regard, the NHS has a champion in Stephen Hawking. While he was on a trip to the USA, Republican politicians criticised the NHS as evil, saying people such as him would not have a chance in the UK. That comment was a remarkably ill-informed hostage to fortune. He responded: "I wouldn't be here today if it were not for the NHS. I have received a large amount of high-quality treatment without which I would not have survived."[36]

Yet, perversely, their argument has some inevitable weight in any system that seeks to make the best overall use of a finite budget, no matter how large that budget may be. We cannot, and should not, deny that.

Certainly, the NHS polarises opinion more than most other things, usually on grounds of quality and value for money. In 1966, Enoch Powell, previously a Minister of Health, succinctly clarified the waters of such financial argument. He wrote that the system of finance in the NHS "endows everyone providing as well as using it with a vested interest in denigrating it."[37] He contrasted this attitude with that in

---

[36] McElroy D (2009). *Stephen Hawking: I Would Not Be Alive Without the NHS. The Telegraph*, 12 August 2009. [online] Available from: http://tinyurl.com/mdpd2z (accessed 9 January 2017).
[37] Powell JE (1966). *A New Look at Medicine and Politics*. London, Pitman.

private medicine, where both the paid and paying make it out to be better than it really is.

Whatever our stance, whether we laud it or criticise it, we should know something about the NHS before casting an opinion. We should find out more than rely on our singular experience of A & E last Saturday after a fall, or the long delay to get an appointment with our GP, or that kindly nurse who was so nice to Jimmy. Something broader and more concrete is needed. Emotion is an inevitable part of care and caring, but unless accompanied by a reasoned, informed argument it can easily impede judgement rather than promote it. That is why I see a historical section as a component of this book.

THE ORIGINS OF THE NHS

So, what is the NHS? Why do we have it? And from where did it come? The story begins at the dawn of the 20th century, decades before the birth of the NHS itself. We must look at that time to understand the reasons why we have it. You may, like me, be surprised how some of the detail of its origins confounds the conventional narrative.

A general summary is straightforward. The NHS began in 1948 as the direct consequence of the National Health Service Act 1946, introduced by Aneurin Bevan and a Labour government. The egalitarian vision underpinning it was that good healthcare should be available to all, regardless of wealth. It was to be truly inclusive and accessible to everyone, even to visitors from abroad. It was to be free at the point of use and funded entirely out of general taxation, rather than through national insurance. Finally, it was to provide care in an equitable manner, according only to need.

Such a summary can be agreed by critics and enthusiasts alike. But there is more to it than that. For example, it could be argued that the Conservative party, rather than Labour, should take the credit – or blame – for inventing the NHS. But then the Liberal party also had a major part to play. So, politically the NHS was very much a tripartite conception. I shall colour in that summary at least a bit more, enough to offer an appropriate backdrop to the rest of the book.

***

Far from being a flash of inspiration given physical form overnight on 5 July 1948, the seeds had been sown and resown over many years by professional bodies and governments of all political persuasions. We can look at the origins of the NHS under a few chronological landmark headings.

THE NATIONAL INSURANCE ACT 1911

Before the NHS, most patients had to pay for their medical care, though there were exceptions. Some local authorities funded hospitals for their ratepayers,[38] and there were health insurance schemes, such as those offered by friendly societies.[39] But it was an uncoordinated hotchpotch of different systems, and conditions were harsh. Annual death rates ran into their thousands for infections such as tuberculosis, meningitis, diphtheria, and pneumonia. Industrial diseases were rife, and 1 in 20 children died before their first birthday.

Scholars can trace the genesis of a national health service back to the 19th century, but for practical purposes, we can take the National Insurance Act of 1911 as our starting point. David Lloyd George, Chancellor of the Exchequer in Asquith's Liberal government, had visited Germany in 1908. He was impressed by Otto von Bismarck's national sickness insurance system which followed the country's

---

[38] In the UK, a ratepayer is a person liable to pay rates. Rates are taxes on land and buildings paid to a local authority.
[39] Friendly societies predated modern insurance companies, but in this context provided a similar function. In essence, for a regular subscription the society would meet the individual's medical costs.

Health Insurance Bill of 1883.[40] Lloyd George declared his intention to follow that example and provide the UK working class with a contributory national insurance scheme. The 1911 Act covered unemployment and illness as part of an array of Liberal social reforms.

Relief provided by the Poor Law had been in existence in one form or another since Tudor times but had been formalised within the Poor Law Amendment Act 1834. However, by the early 20th century such well-intentioned assistance, and its association with the workhouses, was stigmatised and unwelcome. (Even at the beginning of my career, some patients shunned St Edmund's Hospital for older people because of its association with the workhouse four decades previously.) The Liberal government's social welfare reforms of 1906 superseded the Poor Law. The system of workhouses stopped in 1929, and the National Assistance Act abolished the Poor Law in 1948.

Part I of the National Insurance Act 1911 was concerned with sickness insurance. Each worker earning more than £160 a year[41] had to insure himself by contributing 4 pence per week out of his wages,[42] at a time when a pint of beer cost 6 pence; the employer contributed 3 pence, and general taxation provided a further 2 pence. Those on a limited list of manual trades were then eligible to take sick leave at the rate of 10 shillings a week for the first 13 weeks, and 5 shillings a week for the next 13.[43]

They were also given free access to a panel doctor (so called because they were on their panel, later to become a GP's registered list within the NHS), though not necessarily to the cost of medicine. In

---

[40] Otto Leopold, Prince of Bismarck, nicknamed the "Iron Chancellor", became the first Chancellor of a united Germany. A staunch conservative, he created the world's first welfare state, reportedly to drain the support of workers away from the socialists.

[41] Equivalent to £14 600 in 2014, if adjusted according to the RPI.

[42] Equivalent to £1.52 in 2014, if adjusted according to the RPI.

[43] Equating to £45.50 in 2014, if adjusted according to the RPI.

a sign of the times, they were provided with free sanatorium treatment for tuberculosis.

The provision of medical care was patchy both in its content and to whom it applied. For example, it did not cover all trades, nor did it extend to the families of even those workers whom it covered. To a large extent, it was an economic exercise to maintain the country's essential workforce.

Nonetheless, much of the conceptual framework for the NHS arose from this Act. It established the idea of state-funded medical care for lists of registered panels of patients, and the principle of capitation payments to GPs for patients on their panels. It formalised a pre-existing practice of referrals from GP to a hospital specialist, so establishing the GP's gatekeeper role regarding hospital services. And it introduced the "Lloyd George medical record", held by the patient's doctor and, remarkably, to this day still the official paper record of NHS general practice. While the National Health Service Act extended these principles in 1946 and made them universal, it was the 1911 Act that drove into the ground the foundation stakes of the service.

Perhaps the most glaring difference between the two forms of service – those following 1911 and 1948 – is that the 1911 Act was a Bismarckian, national insurance-based system while the NHS that emerged in 1948 was a Bevanite one, funded entirely out of general taxation. We will consider the implications of this fundamental difference later.

During the Second World War, a national Emergency Medical Service was set up to care for civilian injuries. For the first time, doctors and nurses were paid by the state to treat patients in the voluntary hospitals. Though of satisfactory quality, these hospitals were perpetually underfunded and now grew to depend on such state assistance. Even in 1941, in Churchill's war government and five years before Bevan's proposals, the Ministry of Health was considering a comprehensive health service. As a result, the Minister of Health, Ernest Brown, announced his intention to provide a comprehensive hospital service, available to everyone in need.

But few ideas are truly new. Eighty years earlier, the idea of a national hospital service had been raised. In 1861, the Select Committee on Poor Relief received a suggestion of a local hospital treating incurable diseases such as tuberculosis and cancer. Twenty years later, Sir Henry Charles Burdett, financier and philanthropist, consolidated the idea by proposing a geographical district as the catchment area for each large hospital.[44] In reality, one of the main reasons why his coordinated framework of district hospitals did not catch on was the fiercely guarded independence of the large voluntary hospitals.

So, thoughts about at least a national hospital service were being considered 50 years before the 1911 Act. But it was that Act that moved ideas into any form of reality.

THE DAWSON REPORT 1920

However, the greatest effect came in 1920, from the interim report (indeed the only report) of a Consultative Council on Medical and Allied Services to the Ministry of Health, the Dawson Report.[45] In retrospect, that pivotal document can be seen to describe the framework for health services within the UK for the following 90 years. Like so many good ideas, those of the Dawson Report were slow to come to fruition. They failed to gain universal acceptance; the Consultative Council broke up without producing a final report. But

---

[44] Rivett G (undated). *The Development of the London Hospital System, 1823–2015.* [online] Available from: http://tinyurl.com/zc2zpxs (accessed 9 January 2017).
[45] Ministry of Health (1920). *Interim Report on the Future Provision of Medical and Allied Services 1920 (Lord Dawson of Penn).* London, HMSO. Available from: http://tinyurl.com/h8ue9z7 (accessed 9 January 2017).

the vision of the interim report lives on in print and practice. It was only the reforms in 2011 that challenged and removed some of its most fundamental structures, notably the administrative authorities at regional and district levels.

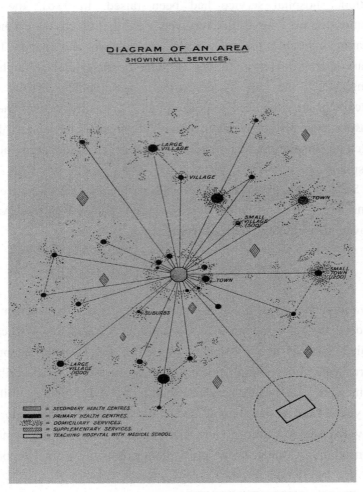

Excerpt from the *Interim Report on the Future Provision of Medical and Allied Services 1920 (Lord Dawson of Penn).*

A short, accessible summary of the Dawson Report is provided by an editorial in the *British Medical Journal* from the day of the report's publication, 28 May 1920.[46] It paints a picture of a remarkably prescient document, one that rejected a wholly salaried service as "the public would be serious losers". Instead, it proposed a mixed contractual structure, with GPs retaining their independence and specialists employed directly and salaried.

It described primary health centres providing additional resources, such as laboratory tests and radiology for GPs, who nonetheless would continue to work from consulting rooms in their homes. To howls of protest from the profession, it described GPs working in groups rather than alone. It included local hospitals (called secondary health centres and providing what we now call secondary – in contrast to primary – care) operating within a district of county size. These would provide a minimum of medicine, surgery, gynaecology, ophthalmology, and ear, nose, and throat. There would be wards for specific conditions – a new idea – staffed by consultants available for referrals from GPs.

The Dawson Report recognised that supplementary services, such as recuperative centres and sanatoria for tuberculosis, would be required:

Primary Centres would ease the work of the Secondary Centres by receiving patients from the Secondary Centres when the acute stage of their illness had passed.[47]

A remark that resonates all too clearly today. Finally, the university hospitals would provide the most specialist services – what today we call tertiary care.

The report's proposed structure recognised the need for an overarching administrative hierarchy. It described health authorities

---

[46] Anon (1920). The report of the Consultative Council. *Br Med J*, 1(3100): 746–747.
[47] Ministry of Health (1920). *Interim Report on the Future Provision of Medical and Allied Services 1920 (Lord Dawson of Penn)*. London, HMSO, Section IV, para 2.

with control of both curative and preventive services, and with an elected local medical advisory council.

There was a debate within the council about paying for the service. Some members argued that all curative and preventive services should be "provided by the health authority free of charge to every individual patient," while others, including the pragmatic Lord Dawson, favoured fitting the existing National Insurance Act organisation into proposals for a mixed economy. He felt many patients were happy to pay for their treatment, and that this would keep the overall cost to the public purse down, as well as maintain standards, thus avoiding the development of a poor service that attracted a bad reputation.

Lord Dawson saw preventive services as being different, of less immediate benefit to the individual, and therefore something for which they would be less inclined to pay. On the other hand, they would be of substantial benefit to the community as a whole. He therefore proposed that preventive services should be provided free to all, and paid for with public funds.

He was a strong advocate of policymakers being assisted by medical expertise, not only at the health authority level but also nationally. He proposed a Consultative Council on Medical and Allied Services for the Minister of Health. Of interest to recent NHS discussion is his related comment, that "it need hardly be said that the ultimate responsibility for decisions would always rest with the Minister."[48]

---

[48] Lord Dawson of Penn (1920). Medicine and the state. The presidential address to the Section of State Medicine in the Brussels Congress of the Royal Institute of Public Health. *Br Med J*, 1(3100): 743–745. [online] Available from: www.ncbi.nlm.nih.gov/pmc/articles/PMC2337416/?page=1 (accessed 9 January 2017).

THE BRITISH MEDICAL ASSOCIATION

And so the country stuttered towards a national health service, though its formal introduction would have to wait until yet another seminal report and the end of the Second World War. Meanwhile, more and more bodies promoted the idea, not least the medical profession itself. The British Medical Association (BMA) published a report in 1938, *A General Medical Service for the Nation*, well before Aneurin Bevan laid his plans before parliament, in which it proposed a comprehensive national health service that should be available to all.

Again before the war, a BMA survey found that 90% of its members favoured a national health service. And in the spring of 1942, the profession's Medical Planning Commission, set up the previous year "to study wartime developments and their effects on the country's medical services both present and future", recommended a centralised, national health service that included hospitals being overseen by regional authorities and GPs working in health centres.[49]

The medical profession's early, persistent advocacy for a national health service contradicts the current beliefs of many. Later, however, the BMA did indeed react, just as it had done to Lord Dawson. As we shall see, it vociferously opposed many aspects of Bevan's proposal, as detailed in his briefing paper for the Cabinet dated 19 January 1948.[50] Among other key matters, the BMA preferred an extension of Lloyd George's Bismarckian national health insurance scheme and the continuing independence of GPs and hospitals.

---

[49] It seemed that by now the profession had got over its fury, 20 years earlier, at Lord Dawson making the same suggestion.

[50] *National Health Service: Attitude of the Medical Profession*. Memorandum by the Minister of Health. The National Archives/The Cabinet Papers 1915–1986. CP (48) 23. [online] Available from: http://tinyurl.com/jz89584 (accessed 9 January 2017).

THE 1942 BEVERIDGE REPORT

The next key figure in this story is William Beveridge, an economist who had advised David Lloyd George about the 1911 Act and later became the director of the London School of Economics and Political Science. In 1941, the government was considering how to rebuild the country after the Second World War, and Beveridge was asked to head an enquiry into social insurance and allied services. His seminal report with the same name was published at the end of 1942 and heralded a welfare state, calling for a fight against what he termed the "five great evils of want, disease, ignorance, squalor and idleness."

He proposed a state-operated system of social security that included a national health service. "Medical treatment covering all requirements will be provided for all citizens by a national health service."[51] His plan was for the system to be implemented after the war.

In broad terms, Lord Dawson, Beveridge, and the BMA were all advocating a universal service, developed from Lloyd George's National Insurance Act. They were joined by Sir Henry Willink, a Conservative and the oft-forgotten Minister of Health in the coalition War Cabinet. Following the Beveridge Report, Willink published a White Paper in February 1944 titled *A National Health Service*. It proposed a fully comprehensive, universal healthcare system that was free of charge and available to everyone irrespective of their ability to pay. Fans of the NHS should give Sir Henry more credit than is usually the case. And its critics on the right of the political spectrum might care to reflect on it originally being the idea of a Conservative government.

When the war ended, Labour defeated the Conservatives in the 1945 general election and Clement Attlee, the new Prime Minister,

---

[51] Rivett G (2012). *Interactive Timeline: the History of NHS Reform*. [online] Available from: http://tinyurl.com/zabntby (accessed 9 January 2017).

proclaimed the introduction of a "cradle to the grave" welfare state based on the Beveridge Report. As we have seen, two of the key components of that report were a national health service and a social security system to underpin every individual. But crucially, while the social security system was built on an expansion of the National Insurance Act 1911, the health service was not. Eventually, it would be funded entirely from general taxation.

ANEURIN BEVAN

The man responsible for introducing the NHS was Aneurin Bevan. While William Beveridge is considered the father of the welfare state, Aneurin Bevan is seen as the chief architect of the NHS. (Poor Lord Dawson seldom gets a mention.) Attlee appointed Bevan Minister of Health in 1945, and his NHS Bill passed into statute in 1946. At a stroke, it nationalised and incorporated nearly 2000 municipal hospitals run by local authorities and over 1300 voluntary ones.

The NHS opened its doors for business on 5 May 1948 and Bevan's name has been pinned above it ever since, despite the Conservatives writing the relevant White Paper shortly before their departure. It seems likely that a government of any description would have introduced one. Nevertheless, it was Bevan who brought it into existence.

The main feature for which he is solely responsible is its method of funding. Against much expert opinion, he was convinced to the point of passion that taxation alone should pay for it. He felt this so strongly that later, in 1951 – by which time he had been moved from the Ministry of Health – he resigned from the Cabinet over the issue of even a few charges being levied on patients. In so doing, he martyred himself for the principles of state-funded, free care for all, and made the funding of the NHS through taxation a political canon that has remained largely untouchable to this day.

Bevan drew two lines of principle in the sand, across which he would not pass. The first was that it must be a comprehensive service free for all; the second that it must be funded out of taxation. He was prepared to negotiate on anything else if it helped deliver a service anchored on those two principles.

As we have seen, with some notable exceptions, the medical profession initially supported the concept. Bevan's difficulties with doctors concerned the detail of how they were to be involved and remunerated, rather than with the principle of a national health service. In his 1998 lecture, "The Bevan legacy", Michael Portillo referred to the obsession and secretiveness of Bevan concerning his proposals.[52] He noted, for example, that Bevan refused to discuss them with the medical profession until after the Bill's first reading in parliament, an extraordinary state of affairs. Confusingly, this contradicts Bevan's speech to the House of Commons in February 1948:

> *I have met the Negotiating Committee itself eight times, three times before the Bill was introduced and – I hope this will not be brought against me – most irregularly I met them three times whilst the Bill was before the Committee.*[53]

As so often in politics, there seem to be at least two sides to the argument, each side cherry-picking appropriate evidence to back a particular case.

What is clear is that Bevan had his work cut out if he was going to get a hostile medical profession on board with his proposals. His intention was to make all specialists and GPs salaried employees of the NHS – the very idea rejected on the patients' behalf by Lord

---

[52] Michael Portillo, Cabinet minister, Conservative government 1992–1997. Portillo M (1998). The Bevan legacy. *BMJ*, 317.
[53] Socialist Health Association (undated). *Bevan's Speech to the House of Commons on the Appointed Day 9 February 1948*. [online] Available from: http://tinyurl.com/hhrkgkz (accessed 9 January 2017).

Dawson in 1920. Private practice was to be banned in the nationalised hospitals. Specialists found this restriction unacceptable.

Bevan was prepared to negotiate, to a point. The agreement he achieved with the specialists was that they could reduce their time contracted to the NHS to have free time to undertake private practice, and that the hospitals would have a small number of private "pay beds" to accommodate this. His subsequent trumpeting that he had "stuffed their mouths with gold" was as characteristic of his brilliant, lilting oratory as it was unhelpful.

GPs were different. For them, the contentious issues were threats to their independence and pensions. They had always been self-employed but were now to be salaried and banned from selling goodwill in their practices when they retired. Goodwill arises when a business is sold at a price greater than the value of its assets, thus providing a form of profit. Traditionally, GPs had sold their practices on retirement and used the goodwill capital to fund their pensions, so the goodwill must have been a quite substantial sum.

They insisted on being independent contractors, arguing that only in this way could they remain their patients' advocates within a state-run system. That may or may not have been disingenuous self-interest at the time, but unfettered patient advocacy is most certainly desirable now – perversely as market forces become prevalent in the NHS.[54]

Bevan finally surmounted these two obstacles with GPs. The two sides agreed to outlaw the sale of goodwill, and that GPs remained independent contractors but able to use the NHS pension scheme. That unique concession for self-employed GPs remains to this day, as does the illegality of selling goodwill within general practice.

Undoubtedly, some BMA leaders adopted a very destructive, hostile posture towards the NHS. One even likened it to being "the

---

[54] A recurring impression woven into the fabric of this book is my belief that the independence of GPs has been a very significant benefit to the development of the NHS and to individual patients.

first step, and a big one, to National Socialism, as practised in Germany"[55] – a particularly vicious, emotive barb delivered so soon after the Second World War. And in a vote held in February 1948 – after the Bill was published but crucially before Bevan addressed their concerns – 40 000 members of the BMA voted against the NHS, with fewer than 5000 expressing their support. That vote is the one conveniently recalled by the profession's critics when saying it rejected the NHS.

Even in hindsight, the doctors' demands seem reasonable. The negotiated settlements mediated by the emollient President of the Royal College of Physicians (RCP), Charles Wilson (later to become Lord Moran), appear pragmatically sensible for all concerned, not least for patients. It seems fair to conclude that both sides wanted an NHS but that the devil was in the detail of its implementation. The critical sticking point was not how the doctors were involved, but Bevan's obduracy in insisting that only taxation should be used for its funding.

When it came to funding the NHS, Bevan had a choice of two theoretical concepts. On the one hand, there was a multiple payer system: government-regulated but private insurance for all, with interventional payments by the state for the financially disadvantaged. This was the one pioneered by Bismarck, adopted by Lloyd George in 1911, favoured by Beveridge in 1942 and by the BMA. Commonly, other countries with nationwide health systems have followed this model, though varying in their detail. The second concept was a single payer system, a service funded entirely by the state. Few other countries have such systems.

But for Aneurin Bevan there was, in reality, no choice; he went with his heart, living out his socialist dream and insisting on a single

---

[55] BBC News, 1 July 1998. *Making Britain Better*. [online] Available from: http://news.bbc.co.uk/1/hi/events/nhs_at_50/special_report/119803.stm (accessed 9 January 2017).

payer system. He carried the day through the power of his oratory and the traction of his principled conviction. While to some extent he developed and enacted the ideas of others, including the BMA and the previous Conservative government, nonetheless Bevan is seen as the architect of the NHS; it was he who turned ideas into reality. History may yet decree that he was an architect whose financial plan contained a fundamental, fatal flaw.

***

One of the most striking things about the NHS is its sheer size. With 1.5 million personnel, it has grown to become the world's largest publicly funded health service, the biggest employer in Europe and among the top five in the world, alongside the Chinese Liberation Army, the United States Department of Defense, and – more surprisingly to me at least – McDonald's and Walmart. Just over half of NHS personnel are clinically qualified, and a further quarter provides close support to clinicians in such roles as healthcare assistants and nursing auxiliaries. Of course, data vary depending on dates and exactly what is measured, but these are reported by the NHS Confederation.[56] I have summarised some of these data here, which apply to the 2014–2015 period.

The NHS employed 149 808 doctors, 314 966 qualified nursing staff and health visitors, 25 418 midwives and 23 066 GP practice nurses.

Planned expenditure for 2015–2016 is £116 574 billion. In 2014, it was on a par with that for each of pensions and welfare; the education budget was 76% of that for health, and the defence budget a mere 42%. UK health expenditure in 2013 was 8.46% of gross domestic product (USA 16.43%, Netherlands 11.12%, Germany 10.98%, France 10.95%, Italy 8.77%). Per capita expenditure in 2013 for the

---

[56] NHS Confederation (2016). *Key Statistics on the NHS*. [online] Available from: http://tinyurl.com/owbegqn (accessed 9 January 2017).

UK (using the purchasing power parity) was $3235 (USA $8713, Netherlands $5131, Germany $4819, France $4124, Italy $3077).

The UK had 2.8 physicians per 1000 people in 2013 (Germany 4.1, Italy 3.9, Spain 3.8, Australia 3.4, France 3.3, New Zealand 2.8, Canada 2.6) and 2.8 hospital beds per 1000 people in 2013 (Germany 8.3, France 6.3, Denmark 3.1, Spain 3.0, New Zealand 2.8).

In 2000, the Labour government argued that the NHS is the cheapest and fairest way to fund healthcare for the entire UK population.[57] Nonetheless, the expenditure figure quoted for 2013 – $3235 per capita – equates to £2273 per year for every person in the UK. Such is the cost of healthcare, but we spend less than many. Of the seven other countries listed, only Italy spent less (yet had 25% more physicians).

It is salutary to compare such comprehensive, unrestricted service to that offered for the same money by a private health insurance policy. Exact comparison is neither possible nor implied here, but the broad thought is interesting. Both systems have the similarity that they spread risk and cost across a defined population.

We might consider the NHS as a health insurance policy unique in its open-ended cover. It is taken out for the entire population yet paid for by its only policyholder, the government, who determines the nature of the cover, yet also – within its annual spending review – decides the size of the premium. No matter what illness I have, when I got it, how long I have it for, the NHS will not renege on its commitment to look after me and all others like me. (How well it meets that responsibility is another matter, but the point here is that unlike any insurance policy, the statutory intention is there.)

Such an arrangement is economically unstable. No insurance company would allow you to take out a policy of unlimited cover for

---

[57] NHS (2000). *The NHS Plan. A Plan for Investment. A Plan for Reform.* Norwich, HMSO. [online] Available from: http://tinyurl.com/z8ys9qd (accessed 9 January 2017).

your entire family, regardless of existing conditions and risk factors, for life and with endless claims, while allowing you to decide the premium. That would be nonsense. In principle, this is the situation for the government and the NHS.

That economic conundrum is why no incoming government can keep its hands off the NHS. It is a service that is hugely expensive, loved by the public, but far from perfect either clinically or economically. So, as night follows day, new governments produce a fresh round of reforms. In 2010, the incoming coalition government followed that tradition, though compared to past examples its proposals were especially vigorous, despite neither the Conservatives nor the Liberal Democrats having included such plans in their election manifesto.

Over the decades, the organisational shape of the NHS has reflected these various changes, jerking from one engineered mutation to the next like a poorly controlled puppet. The most far-reaching took place in 1990 with the introduction of an NHS internal market, but none comes close to matching the visionary impact of Lord Dawson in 1920, Beveridge in 1942, or Bevan in 1946. The most accessible, authoritative review of these changes is by Geoffrey Rivett, and is freely available on the World Wide Web (WWW).[58] His writing satisfies all but the most particular student of the NHS. Here we will just sketch in some of the broad principles.

***

To appreciate how NHS organisation has evolved requires understanding that, in 1948, it was divided into three parts: (1) hospital services, managed by 400 hospital management committees that were themselves answerable to the 14 regional hospital boards (RHBs); (2) community services, the responsibility of local

---

[58] Rivett GC (undated). *National Health Service History*. [online] Available from: www.nhshistory.net/ (accessed 9 January 2017).

authorities; and (3) primary care: GPs, opticians, pharmacists, and dentists were independent contractors to the NHS.

GPs were contracted to the NHS to provide "all necessary care" for a defined list of registered patients. For that, they received remuneration according to a contract negotiated nationally between the BMA and the government. Predominantly, this consisted of capitation payments proportional to the number of patients registered with them. Local executive councils undertook the administration of general practice, administering contracts and payments, and maintaining registers of each GP's patients.

Initially, the hospitals were far from a comprehensive, cohesive service, despite the RHBs. It was Enoch Powell who, as Health Secretary, placed a logical structure on the rambling mishmash he inherited. His 1962 Hospital Plan echoed some of Henry Burdett's proposals from 80 years before, introducing geographical health districts serving populations of roughly 125 000 people, each with its own district general hospital (DGH). Although it was slow in implementation – largely because of high building costs for the new DGHs – the Hospital Plan was a blueprint for the hospital service thereafter.

From there the service became framed around a hierarchy of distinct geographic areas: countries, regions, areas (briefly), and districts, with statutory authorities charged with providing for the relevant populations. That structure demonstrates all too clearly how the NHS is more than a personal medical service. It is something far more complex; its intention is to be equitable and population-based. To plagiarise an apt phrase from Kaiser Permanente, a US Health Maintenance Organisation, the NHS is concerned with "population care, one patient at a time."

BRINGING THE NHS UP TO DATE: 1974–2005

> *We trained hard, but it seemed that every time we were beginning to form up into teams, we would be reorganised. I was to learn later in life that we tend to meet any new solution by reorganising; and a wonderful method it can be for creating the illusion of progress while producing confusion, inefficiency, and demoralisation.*
>
> British army barrack room wall, the late 1940s. Commonly attributed to Charlton Ogburn Jr (1957) and usually misattributed to Gaius Petronius Arbiter, 27–66 AD.

THE PHASE OF CONSENSUS ADMINISTRATION: 1974–1985

The first major reorganisation of the service took place in 1974. In an echo of 1948, it was planned in outline by the Conservatives but implemented by the incoming Labour government of Harold Wilson. Fourteen RHAs made up the top layer with 90 subordinate area health authorities to manage hospitals and community services, and a corresponding set of 90 family practitioner committees (FPCs), new organisations that administered primary care in place of the previous executive councils. Finally, at a local level, hospitals continued to be managed by the district health authorities (DHAs).

The accompanying *Grey Book* characterised the underlying philosophy of this reorganisation; a large, national document encompassing everything on how to run the hospitals and community care. An instruction manual, setting out every detail of the aims and functions of the service, it reflected purist, bureaucratic thinking.

Primary care was different. GPs had a *Statement of Fees and*

Allowances, initially produced in 1966 but reissued in 1972 as a loose-leaf A5[59] *Red Book*. It was a set of contractual regulations for these independent contractors, rather than the *Grey Book*'s instructional blueprint for the rest of the service.

Below regional level, primary care sat on one side of a significant gulf, and hospital and community health services (HCHS) sat on the other. This primary–secondary care divide has been an enduring obstacle to cohesive patient care within the NHS, and one that has yet to be satisfactorily bridged.

Within that structure, from 1974 to 1985 each hospital was run by a triumvirate of the senior hospital administrator, senior nurse, and a senior doctor. In the lexicon of the NHS, hospitals were now termed units, and this trio made up the unit management team. It was accountable to its DHA, where there was a similar trio, the district management team. In the same way, the district answered to the RHA and its regional management team. Armed with the *Grey Book* that described how to run the service, the whole thing was very logical and astonishingly bureaucratic.

At each level, the members of the management team were equal partners practising consensus management. All three had to agree on any decision. For some this was very empowering, particularly if the members had a shared vision, got on well, and had similar principles. In other areas, it was a recipe for organisational paralysis and stagnation.

The relevance of general practice at that time to politicians and the rest of the NHS was as a collateral gatekeeper to the dominant and expensive hospitals. Other than that, it was not seen as so very different from the other primary care contractors – community pharmacists, opticians, and dentists.

All primary care contractors were the responsibility of FPCs. As autonomous, independent contractors they could not be directly

---

[59] A standard European size of paper measuring 210 × 148 mm.

managed. All an FPC could do was to administer them. As we saw earlier, this role was further hampered by the lack of a clear description of what a GP was meant to do. Some described it as the John Wayne principle: "a GP has got to do what a GP has got to do." How do you administer that?

In reality, the role of the FPC was simply to pay GPs for what they decided to do. GPs could have done anything, provided it conformed to the opaque rules and regulations set down in their Red Book.

The key point here is that the organisational hallmark for the NHS between 1974 and 1985 was bureaucracy. The strategic intent was to create efficiency and order through consensus management within the HCHS, and administration within primary care.

THE PHASE OF ACCOUNTABLE MANAGEMENT

Sparks began to fly in 1985 following the publication of another seminal document, the Griffiths Report. Sir Roy Griffiths had been chair of the retailer Sainsbury's and in the early 1980s was asked by the new government of Margaret Thatcher to study the NHS and advise how to make it better. He wanted to see single, accountable officers. He wanted to know with which individual the buck stopped. After his recommendations in 1985, the NHS reorganised again, moving from administrators to chief executives; to accountability, command, and control. Out went the consensus trio of an administrator, senior nurse, and senior doctor, each with the power of veto over any decision, and with their rather woolly, collective responsibility. In came chief executives, personal accountability, and direct management hierarchies.

The Griffiths Report was hugely influential and still echoes today. It recommended health authorities should involve clinicians more closely in the management process. They should participate fully in decisions about priorities in the use of resources. Boards should obtain the experience and views of patients and the community about local services.

Griffiths noted that the NHS still lacked any real continuous evaluation of its performance; it lacked incentives to change, and he wanted these introduced. His central concern was for providing a high-quality service to the individual patient, and his methods were those of centralist management. As such, between 1986 and 1990 the service was increasingly a managed one. Nothing emphasised this change more than the introduction of a new managerial incentive – the performance target.[60]

FPCs were not exempt from change. General management arrived for them in 1989 with a change to become more testosterone-fuelled family health service authorities (FHSAs). Help was at hand in the form of a new GP contract that introduced at least some specific requirements and targets.

THE RISE OF GENERAL PRACTICE

In 1988, following pressure from her Chancellor Nigel Lawson, Margaret Thatcher turned her gaze on the NHS. The Chancellor had insisted that he would only provide more money for the service if it demonstrated financial effectiveness. She ordered a review, which she led herself. This secretive process went on for some months, largely behind closed doors.

When Kenneth Clarke took over as Secretary of State in 1989, he worked with her to create an internal market in the health service. An internal market is one operating within an organisation whereby it decouples the composite sections, which then trade their services with each other.

---

[60] Many blame these on Tony Blair's Labour government. In fact, that accolade should go to the Griffiths Report and the government of Margaret Thatcher, though Labour considerably expanded their number.

The internal market divided the NHS between "providers" of services – most obviously the hospitals in secondary care – and "purchasers" of services – most obviously the health authorities that, until then, had not only planned local services but also managed the hospitals. It mainly ignored providers of primary care.

Kenneth Clarke also introduced the idea of larger general practices being able to negotiate a budget to fund their staff, administration, and prescribing costs and purchase 15–20% of the secondary care used by their patients. So, initially, the health authorities purchased 100% of the services for non-fundholding practices and 80% of those for fundholders.

The idea of the market was that dividing providers from purchasers would mean that market competition, for the first time, was to be used to raise standards, reduce waiting lists, bring the selection of services closer to the patient, and provoke cost efficiencies.

For the NHS, this was a shift in its tectonic plates, and it would never be the same again. The omnipotent, resource-devouring hospitals now found themselves within a commercial setting. Others would decide whether or not to buy their services. In theory, the purchasers might choose to buy everything elsewhere, leaving the hospital with no patients to treat and faced with closure. In practice, for political reasons, no such thing would have been allowed to happen. But even in a pseudomarket, a small change in service provision could significantly affect the viability of clinical departments, meaning hospitals had to respond.

The internal market provoked fierce debate. It was certainly remarkable to introduce such extensive changes without trial. The government had chosen to proceed without any evaluated pilot studies despite calls for an incremental introduction, not only from Professor Alain Enthoven, the American academic who first proposed an NHS internal market in 1984, but also from the House of Commons Health

Select Committee. Sir Ian Gilmour, a member of the Cabinet at the time, albeit one to the left of the party, wrote in his memoirs:

> *Dogma, however, overrides common sense, and such things as pilot studies were wholly alien to Thatcherism: they betrayed uncertainty of conviction. The Thatcherite refusal to test the plan by ordering pilot studies was fully comprehensible; any studies would almost certainly have shown that the reforms were undesirable. In consequence pilot studies would have been too big a risk.*[61]

Some might argue that the progressive implementation was itself a form of piloting, but that would be naïve. The government's strategy was abundantly clear; it intended to allocate budgets to as many practices as possible. There was never any doubt about that, so pilot studies were unnecessary. The phased introduction was merely for logistical and political reasons. To counter GP hostility, it had to appear to be an option.

Kenneth Clarke's original idea contravened some of the principles of the NHS and was undesirable in its long-term implications. As we shall see later, in practical terms it was also unsustainable, but it provided a powerful kick to doctors and health authorities to produce viable and beneficial variations and alternatives. Given those modifications (discussed further in the chapter titled "Reforming the Reforms") the Thatcher/Clarke market strategy has remained unchallenged ever since, whatever the government in power, though there have been changes to the operational details.

The incoming government in May 1997 introduced yet another major reorganisation, and over time dramatically extended the market economy. Initially, it fulfilled a manifesto commitment and abolished fundholding, but then reintroduced it in a much improved and less contentious form, displaying linguistic dexterity in calling it practice-

---

[61] Gilmour I (1992). *Dancing with Dogma: Britain Under Thatcherism.* London, Simon & Shuster Ltd, p. 159.

based commissioning. Strategic health authorities replaced the RHAs and, at the district level, DHAs and FHSAs were combined into new authorities.

All this revolving of bureaucratic doors continued to spew out new bodies with different functions and shapes, but at a local level these essentially did much the same task of organising the service. And so, an interesting dichotomy within the NHS continued. On the surface, the process of clinical care for the individual patient remained virtually unchanged, while beneath the waves politicians, civil servants, and managers busied themselves endlessly repositioning the boulders on the seabed. Many impartial observers would predict little obvious benefit for individual patients from these submerged, energy-sapping boulder movements, and they would be right.

The Blair government gathered the best strands of GP involvement that emerged during the Thatcher years, from both those with and without budgets, and blended them into primary care groups (PCGs). For legislative reasons, if no other, these were a subsidiary component, a subcommittee, of the health authorities, which still held the local budget. Most importantly, they involved multiple practices, thus reducing, if not eliminating, many of the most significant faults of the original single-practice fundholding scheme. When the necessary legislation eventually passed into law, PCGs evolved into primary care trusts (PCTs), and they became statutory authorities, holding and responsible for their budget.

PCTs could now replace health authorities, something politicians would proudly trumpet as removing various managerial and administrative departments from the service. In fact, their rhetoric exceeded reality. Overall, the tasks of PCTs were much the same as those of the old health authorities, so inevitably they re-employed many of the health authority staff to work for them, often even doing their old jobs. Nonetheless, this strategy continued the perpetual, dichotomous quest of governments. On the one hand, it was to trim managerial fat from the burgeoning body of the NHS, and on the other, to reposition decision-making and accountability on the shoulders of local clinicians and managers, and therefore away from government. Who of us has not heard a government minister explain that, as they had passed decision-making to local groups, they could no longer comment on X, Y, or Z? How convenient. So, if you do not like something, blame your local doctors, the ones you trust with your confidential, personal care.

There were undoubted successes for all the additional money made available to the NHS by the Labour government. Perhaps the most striking were the reductions in a hospital's waiting times from months, even years, to a matter of weeks. But this was not the market at work. Such genuine benefits for patients followed the imposition of enforced targets and increased funding, rather than a response to market forces. Once those relaxed in 2011, waiting times started to rise once more despite an unchanged market.

Another success was the introduction of the Quality and Outcomes Framework (QOF) for general practice. Again, this involved targets set nationally rather than change through a market economy. But the plethora of imposed hoops through which managers and clinical staff were to jump was stifling. People were overwhelmed, and there was no time left for local initiatives and innovation. Inevitably, morale sagged. The *Grey* and *Red Books* from the years of consensus management and administration had gone, replaced with centralist micromanagement complete with dictates, accountability to higher authorities, and a barrowload of sticks and carrots.

It would have been better to establish a few essential, national, key objectives, agreed and endorsed by representatives from all the bodies concerned. Those could then be focused on as national priorities while leaving local communities time and resources to determine their other needs, preferences, and plans. As Griffiths had said, it was not for government to engage in the day-to-day management of the NHS. It seems no one listened to that bit.

There have been other changes in the last 20 years, but the direction of travel remains that set out by Roy Griffiths, Margaret Thatcher, and Kenneth Clarke. GPs – the pit-face generalists – have had an ever-increasing influence as planners and managers of local services for their patients.

No one pursued this strategy more vigorously than the Labour Secretary of State for Health, Alan Milburn. Professor Enthoven himself is reported to have described the Thatcher/Clarke implementation of his ideas as comparatively timid compared to that of Blair/Milburn, whose vision of a "bold, wide-open market" he admired. So Enthoven, the originator of the idea behind the Conservatives' NHS internal market – an innovation opposed by Alan Milburn when in Opposition – was here saying that the Conservatives did not go far enough, and that ironically only Alan Milburn, now in power, had developed the concept properly!

The shift in work, influence, and power from hospitals to general practice has been more striking and significant than the frequent shuffling of the chess pieces of bureaucracy. It has fuelled the most important changes in the NHS, and it reached its logical conclusion in the Health and Social Care Act 2012.

THE HEALTH AND SOCIAL CARE ACT 2012

The structure of the NHS now looked entirely different. At the time of writing, it is the current organisational structure of the NHS, and therefore not only beyond the time span of this book but descriptions are also readily accessible elsewhere.[62]

---

[62] NHS Choices (undated). *The NHS in England.* [online] Available from: www.nhs.uk/NHSEngland (accessed 9 January 2017).

Much of the previous layered hierarchy disappeared. Gone were NHS authorities at regional and district levels. The local planning, procurement, and contracting functions for secondary care were now the responsibility of CCGs, which replaced PCTs on 1 April 2013. CCGs are clinically led statutory NHS bodies responsible for the planning and commissioning of healthcare services for their local area. There are now a little over 200 CCGs in England.

Another change was that local government once more became involved, assuming responsibility for community services and public health as it had done before 1974. It also had the responsibility, through its new health and wellbeing board, for developing and overseeing a local joint strategic needs assessment and strategy. This document is the means by which local authorities, public health, social services, CCGs, local hospitals, and organisations will undertake the strategic planning, coordination, and accountability of services for their local population. This theoretically attractive idea echoed the work done in the Northamptonshire Health Authority 10 years earlier, though I doubt government policymakers had ever read our report *A Sense of Place* (see the chapter titled "Working with the Authorities").

Leaving aside financial and probity imponderables, there are other issues of significance. As the years roll by, will those GPs who are rising to the management surface carry on in that role? Will there be enough of them? After all, the logic behind CCGs is that commissioning will be better if it makes use of the knowledge of local GPs and their understanding of patients' needs. As the initial excitement fades and the pressures of economic reality bear down, most clinicians in the past have tended to melt away from management. District medical officers in the administrative phase of the NHS, chief executives in its early accountable management phase, and even individual fundholders or locality commissioning GPs have all tended to do that.

The consensus, strategic view of most clinicians has always been to leave management to managers. It seems inevitable that the CCGs will subcontract much of their commissioning work to external parties. But to whom? There has been much interest already from large organisations outside the NHS. The consequences of such a move are unknown, but the stakes are high. In 2013–2014, NHS England allocated £63.4 billion to CCGs for purchasing services for their populations, and a further £1.3 billion for their operational costs.

***

So, what has changed with all those structural reorganisations to make GPs so pivotal? First, policymakers have at last come to realise that GPs are the hub of the NHS. Most of the contacts between patients and the NHS occur in primary care. Hospital care usually starts and ends in general practice and – of greatest importance to governments – one way or another, GPs disburse most of the NHS budget spent directly on patient care.

To most impartial observers it then follows that the NHS needs to manage GPs and their practices, especially regarding their referrals to expensive hospital care, and in their use of the pressured NHS prescribing budget. If the GP gatekeeper role is a commonplace for discussion, less often mentioned is the need to lift the quality of the care GPs provide within their practices.

The emotional shift policymakers need to make is not yet complete. They see the problem and the opportunity, but still miss a key component of the solution. They accept the importance of GPs to NHS expenditure, and the consequential need to have greater control over them. They also recognise the need to increase the service quality in general practice. But what they have yet to grasp is the need for practices to have the necessary resources to do this.

There is considerable international evidence linking strong primary care with better overall health outcomes. For example, Dr Barbara

Starfield, a highly respected American academic and paediatrician, studied primary care extensively within both the NHS and other international communities. She showed that money invested in primary care produces better health outcomes at less cost and with a better patient experience than spending the same money on hospital services. Her work was welcome empirical support for common sense. The developing world recognises it, where opportunity costs are seen to matter. But somehow, it is lost on policymakers here and elsewhere in countries that see themselves as the "developed" world. We continue to pour resources disproportionally into secondary and tertiary care, the homes of clinical television drama and human emotion.

Our politicians respond to public opinion, represented so powerfully by the media. Within that world, special care units will always trump immunisation programmes. Even before the NHS, some recognised this. In 1845, the new Royal Victoria Dispensary offered vaccinations for free. Preventive medicine was a common good, usually of no immediate benefit to the patient but ultimately of benefit to all. In 1920, Lord Dawson took the same view, advocating public funding of preventive health measures. Crudely, it was a cost-effective use of public money. The economic theory concerning healthcare will always have to bend to emotional forces, but hopefully not to the point that it breaks.

The matter of management and quality control within general practice is difficult, given that GPs are still commonly self-employed, independent contractors. But here the 2012 reforms contained a master stroke of genius. It completed a major quality improvement circle in a politically astute manner. GP commissioning under the 2012 Act was the ultimate expression of collective responsibility, for regulations required every practice to be part of a CCG. If these groups were to manage their corporate budget effectively, then inevitably they would apply pressures on their members regarding consistent clinical behaviour.

In this way, peer accountability among these technically independent contractors would raise clinical standards within the practices while also managing their use of secondary care. There is evidence from GP cooperative groups in the past, such as the multifund and locality commissioning groups (LCGs) discussed in the chapter titled "Reforming the Reforms", that such peer pressure works and avoids the interference from non-clinical managers that the professional, clinical psyche finds so distressing. (The chapter describes just how such changes in clinical behaviour occurred because of collaboration between clinicians between 1993 and 1994.)

And there is a third, crucial and empowering point behind the ascent of general practice. The arrival of microcomputers[63] in the 1980s has allowed it to encompass preventive care for its populations of patients, and to take most of the management of ongoing conditions away from hospitals.

---

[63] It is only microcomputers that have been used in general practice since the 1980s; accordingly, the "micro" is usually dropped. Therefore, through the book I use the words microcomputer and computer interchangeably, unless I say I am specifically referring to mainframe or minicomputers.

THE FOUR CORNERSTONES

The changes that led to the current, pivotal position of general practice began in the 1970s, but why, and what were they? There was no single cause. The previous chapter touched on the political decisions, but three other things also stirred the primeval soup of the NHS to create what we might call modern general practice.

THE BMA

We have already seen that general practice was a distinctly poor relation of the hospitals. It was underfunded, seen as an inferior career, and had no professional structure of its own. By 1965, it was in the gutter; morale was so low there were calls for revolt. The General Medical Services Committee (GMSC) of the BMA produced a pamphlet, *A Charter for the Family Doctor Service*, and demanded its use as the basis for a new national contract for GPs. It is said to have been written by five senior GPs over a weekend in Brighton, but it echoed an earlier document, *Our Blueprint for the Future*, written and published the previous year by the Medical Practitioners' Union (MPU).[64] That document was never publicly recognised by the GMSC – a sad example of professional plagiarism by the large from the small. There can be no doubt that the GMSC considered *Our Blueprint for the Future*, for within the archives of the BMA I found a copy neatly bound into the minutes of the relevant GMSC committee meeting.

The MPU remains a much smaller organisation than the BMA, but it has always been a creative, left-wing think tank within the profession. It formed as the Medico-Political Union in 1914 but

---

[64] Medical Practitioners' Union (1964). *Our Blueprint for the Future.* London, MPU.

changed its name to MPU in 1922. It opposed, and was an alternative to, the BMA. It is now within the Unite trade union.[65] It seems its inspirational document was adapted by the Brighton five that weekend, and then published as the BMA's famous Charter, but the MPU deserves credit for its original work.

The full GMSC agreed on the four-page Charter and presented it within a few weeks to Kenneth Robinson, the Minister of Health. He seemed reluctant to take either the BMA or its demands seriously. That may be because of the document's miniscule length, something unusual to politicians and civil servants who seem to assess reports not so much by their content as their weight. That was a bad mistake, for the GMSC was deadly serious. It asked for signed but undated letters of resignation from all the 21 489 GPs in the UK. It received 17 580, representing 82% of the total. All the GMSC would have to do was date the letters, hand them in en masse, and the NHS would be without most of its GPs. For good. Suddenly without its engine, it would slew around in the water to an almost immediate dead stop.[66]

Politically this was an overwhelming mandate for the GMSC negotiators. It dwarfed the much better-known actions of Arthur Scargill and the coal miners in 1984–1985. You can stockpile coal, but not healthcare. In any case, this was not a threat to strike for 2–5 days, as was the case of junior hospital doctors in 2016, but the resignation of four-fifths of all GPs from the NHS. To borrow from a Black Friday slogan: once doctors have gone, they have gone. It is

---

[65] Unite the Union, commonly known as Unite, is a British and Irish trade union formed on 1 May 2007, by the merger of Amicus and the Transport and General Workers' Union. It is the largest trade union in the UK and Ireland.

[66] GPs were not as callous as this implies. With every letter of resignation, the BMA collected a significant sum of money with which, if necessary, it would start up an alternative health system for patients. The money was not required, but I have been unable to establish whether the doctors ever got it back.

hard to imagine a more potent industrial negotiating hand by anyone within the UK.

And because of that, and unlike the threats and strikes of the miners and junior doctors, it worked. By the middle of March 1965, Kenneth Robinson accepted the Charter as the basis for negotiating a new contract introduced the following year. Ever since, politicians have been wary of the exceptional bargaining clout of a united medical profession.

A *Charter for the Family Doctor Service* was an extraordinary document in its clarity, brevity, and compass. It was a much improved, succinct version of *Our Blueprint for the Future* though adding little original to its content. It called for doctors to be able to work in suitable premises, have adequate equipment and ancillary help, work in close contact with professional colleagues, have access to modern facilities and hospital beds, have time to look after patients properly and keep up to date with professional knowledge.

Even in retrospect, that appears a coherent group of requirements. Our difficulty is in appreciating that these things did not exist before the Charter. There can be no doubt that it was indeed a blueprint, and one for the biggest change in general practice that has ever taken place. Its legacy shines throughout the NHS to this day, to the benefit of patients everywhere, for more than any other set of demands it established the physical infrastructure of modern general practice.

THE COLLEGE OF GENERAL PRACTITIONERS

Another cornerstone of modern general practice was the creation of the CGP 14 years earlier. A group of frustrated, high-minded GPs led by Dr John Hunt established it in 1952. In seeking to improve the quality of their practices, Hunt and his colleagues adopted a strategy of education and research to develop standards of care. The BMA had advocated formal training in its 1950 Cullen Report, but it was the CGP in the 1960s and 1970s that took up the challenge and pioneered vocational training. In 1976, the government made such training mandatory for all entering general practice.

As the organising and authorising body for training practices, the CGP could impose its ideas on them. The manner in which these practices complied with the rules demonstrates how a central requirement that facilitates the desired goal effects change within fiercely independent practices. It was a lesson not lost on the Department of Health (DoH) and its political masters.

In later chapters, we look further at the important efforts of the RCGP[67] in raising standards of research, quality, education, and professional standing. But for now, we will return to the Charter negotiations in 1965.

MIND THE GAP

No matter the overall excellence of the Charter, something was missing from the 1966 contract that followed. Its five authors almost certainly had no formal management training between them and, in any case, they were first and foremost elected servants of the membership of the BMA. It was not for them to throw a spanner into their own wheel.

With far less excuse, the government's negotiators also missed the gap. The groundbreaking contract failed to provide adequate incentives and accountability to ensure that patient care was improved. By implementing the Charter's demands, it facilitated improvements among the committed good while failing to do much to lift the standards of the uncommitted poor. Providing opportunities for improved working conditions, education, and facilities were not enough to raise quality standards across the board, any more than

---

[67] The CGP was formed in 1952. It aquired its royal prefix (RCGP) in 1967 and royal charter in 1972.

placing water before horses makes them drink. Some will and some will not – it is up to the horse.

The RCGP made progressive efforts to raise quality standards among its members, though its attitude might be described as the gentle approach of a seemly, academic club rather than as full-on commitment. Globally, its efforts were ineffective – at least in the short term. General practice persistently failed to adopt the managerial attitude others expected of a profession charged with self-regulation.[68] That was unacceptable to the Conservative government of Margaret Thatcher, with its enthusiasm for competition and cost savings within the NHS as advocated by Sir Roy Griffiths. Kenneth Clarke, Secretary of State for Health, imposed another contract on an unwilling profession, shifting the focus of income from capitation to performance. For the first time, GPs had specified performance objectives and targets linked to remuneration.

In anything, it is the requirement to achieve objectives that instils a need for management, and efficient management needs information. The effects of the new contract resulted in a rapid escalation in the development of GP information systems, which conveniently could now be computer-based. Whether a proud profession with altruistic leanings likes to admit it or not, rewarded targets are powerful motivating forces for change and for improving standards. Any parent knows that. Prophets within the profession had long opined that if it did not take charge itself of raising standards, then others would. Well, it did not, and they did.

The considerable developments in general practice between 1956 and 1974 reflected two major drivers – and the profession instigated both. The most important was the BMA Charter, the other the educational and standard-setting role of the RCGP. Both helped the

---

[68] At its very best, the RCGP's efforts only addressed its members – less than half of all GPs at that time – and many of those were among the more progressive anyhow.

motivated to develop their practices to high standards, but did little to raise standards of clinical care where intrinsic motivation was lacking. The result was a fragmentation of quality, despite the profession's own inadequate attempts at self-regulation.

This leads to the third key driver for change. To a 1989 Thatcher government seeking improved overall standards and increased value for money, the obvious conclusion was to impose its definition of standards via a radically altered, and prescriptive, contract for GPs.

To these three national initiatives we must add a fourth major factor. It was the availability of computers that enabled the imposed contract, which resulted in a sea change in preventive medicine and the management of long-term conditions, and which facilitated measurement within practices, both clinical and managerial.

***

These then are the four national cornerstones of modern NHS general practice: the Charter, the RCGP, contract targets, and computers. Against that background, we can now narrow our focus to a single practice, and consider its operational framework, information systems, buildings, personnel, and management. The following chapters deal with each of these in turn.

PART THREE

THE THREE LIMBS OF CLINICAL PRACTICE

We have a problem. We make an appointment (eventually). We see a doctor whom we may or may not have seen before, and to whom we may need to return later to see how we are getting on. Sometimes they take our blood pressure, sometimes they suggest a flu jab, or that our children have the necessary immunisations.

If we have something serious, the doctor will refer us to the hospital, where (eventually) we will be seen by a specialist, whom we have probably never seen before.

For many that might be a rough sketch of our experience of general practice. But again, a broader knowledge will give us more informed views. It is not that simple now, even if it was in the past. Part Three describes the three interlocking areas of clinical care within modern general practice.

ACUTE CARE

The good physician treats the disease; the great physician treats the patient who has the disease.

William Osler[69]

The term acute care is confusing. To most lay people it suggests severe, as in "he was in acute pain". And things are not helped by many of the DGHs of the recent past now being rebadged as acute hospitals, or acute trusts. In 2010, the King's Fund defined acute illness as being of short duration, and of minor or major significance.

So, a case of tonsillitis is an acute problem, a routine review of diabetes is not, but a person with diabetes who also has tonsillitis may well be. This description is not tiresome pedantry on my part, but rather an attempt to explain a confusing term. Within a practice, the care received by patients is divided into three broad areas: acute care, preventive care, and the management of ongoing conditions – usually termed chronic disease management. As the following two chapters show, acute consultations differ both clinically and in their organisation from the other two areas.

Does the nomenclature matter? To patients, usually not, but for practices the clinical and organisational differences are important. When we have a new problem and want to see someone, or later – when we return for review to ensure our recovery – that is acute care. We arrange the consultation; it is our decision.

A striking difference between primary care and hospitals is that we can decide to go to a GP, dentist, chemist, or optician, but cannot do

---

[69] Sir William Osler was a Canadian physician and one of the four founding professors of the distinguished Johns Hopkins Hospital in the USA.

that with hospitals, whether they call themselves acute or not. With only a few exceptions, to go to hospital we need an invitation. One is the A & E department, for this very reason seen by some as part of primary care and unsurprisingly used as such by some patients. Another is the labour ward, though understandably midwives prefer us to have booked in advance.

Even emergency admissions to a hospital should usually be preceded by a phone call from a referring doctor, as illustrated by the man described with a reinforcing bar stuck through his head (see the chapter titled "Training to Be a GP").

THE HISTORY OF ACUTE CARE

Of course, medicine has changed over time. A century or two ago, the scourge was infections, with pneumonia, smallpox, dysentery, meningitis, and diphtheria all rife, and with no effective vaccination or immunisation programmes, and no antibiotics. Now infection is a less significant factor; antibiotics treat many potentially life-threatening conditions (such as bacterial meningitis or pneumonia) and others are countered (measles, tetanus, polio) or eradicated (smallpox) by vaccination programmes.[70] On the other hand, cancers and the degenerative sequelae of ageing have assumed a more dominant position. Dementia is reaching for the top of the list of causes of death in the UK.

Many years ago, a patient gave me a textbook of medicine published in 1830. It was written by William Buchan MD, of the RCP in Edinburgh, and offers a fascinating insight into medical practice at that time – the time of the Poor Law and my earliest predecessors, Branwhite Spurgin and William Barr.

---

[70] Infection is once more becoming a threat because bacteria are becoming resistant to antibiotics. They are assisted in this process by the inappropriate use of antibiotics for minor and frequently viral conditions, and the widespread use of antibiotics in agriculture.

101 · PRACTICE MATTERS

It explains in great detail the treatment of such prevalent conditions as "the croup". Croup is a form of upper respiratory infection that typically affects young children below the age of three; it is characterised by a striking, dog-like bark that alarms both patient and parent. Now, it is often treated with a single dose of steroids, but in the early days of my practice, a seriously steamy atmosphere worked wonders, particularly if accompanied by distraction and reassuring smiles from adults. For our own children, we found a plastic Wendy house[71] worked a treat, a do-it-yourself echo of the steam tents used at that time in hospitals. We filled it with steam from a kettle before adding toys, a favourite teddy bear, drinks, and patient. We then offered hearty, smiling encouragement through the doorway or windows. Following our success, I recommended it to patients. Each winter before adopting my Wendy house treatment, I admitted several patients with croup for steam tent treatment. Afterwards, I only ever felt the need to admit one.

But medical practice was far more complicated for Dr Buchan in 1830. He mentions steam, though almost as an aside in more than two pages devoted to the croup. He places much greater emphasis on the immediate immersion of the patient's feet in warm water and applying 3–6 leeches according to size (whether of the patient or the leech is not specified) to the sick child's throat to bleed them. He also advises the encouragement of vomiting by the use of emetics:

Upon the first attack of the disease, vomiting, immediately after bleeding, seems to be of considerable use, and sometimes suddenly removes the disease.[72]

---

[71] This is a toy house large enough for children to play in. It is named after the house built around Wendy in JM Barrie's play *Peter Pan*.
[72] Buchan W (1830). *Domestic Medicine or, a Treatise on the Prevention and Cure of Diseases by Regimen and Simple Medicines*. London, Lewis, p. 348.

I am not surprised; the patient would do anything to avoid more of such treatment! I think our toys and drinks in a familiar, play steam tent were a safer distraction than leeches crawling around your neck and induced vomiting. But then I suppose I would.

But Dr Buchan is not finished yet. He provides an apothecary's pharmacopoeia to be tried, including camphor, vitriolated zinc, oxymel of squills,[73] salt of tartar, calomel,[74] blistering plasters around the neck and shoulders, and acetated water of ammonia:

> *In addition, the child may frequently take a tablespoonful of the following mixture: milk of gum ammoniacum[75] three ounces, hyssop[76] of pennyroyal[77] water two ounces, oxymel of squills three drachms,[78] syrup of marsh-mallows and of white poppies of each an ounce, mix them together.*

And so his advice goes on, though present-day physicians may be particularly alarmed to read the recommendation to prescribe "tincture of opium, in doses of five, six to eight drops, given every two hours until sleep." Indeed, opium is an excellent sedative, but it also suppresses the respiratory system, which with croup is already struggling.

---

[73] Oxymel was a medicinal drink or syrup made of vinegar and honey, sometimes administered with other ingredients, such as squills (an extract of the bulb of the squill, a coastal Mediterranean plant of the lily family, which although poisonous has medicinal and other uses).

[74] Also known as mercurous chloride, a white powder formerly used as a purgative.

[75] A gum resin exuded from the stem of the perennial herb *Dorema ammoniacum*. It was used for the treatment of bronchial affections, and for treating asthma and chronic colds.

[76] An aromatic plant of the mint family; the bitter minty leaves are used in cooking and herbal medicine.

[77] Another small-leaved plant of the mint family, also used in herbal medicine.

[78] A unit of weight formerly used by apothecaries, equivalent to 60 grains or one-eighth of an ounce.

And there I was, thinking that medicine had become more complicated.

ACUTE CARE IN PRACTICE

Part of the excitement and challenge of general practice is that you always must be prepared to deal with the unexpected and unusual acute case. One Sunday afternoon when on call, I was busy in the kitchen, bottling a promising white wine home brew. The phone went; it always did at the wrong moment. An anxious father explained that his teenage daughter had a pain in her tummy and could I visit? Of course; I would be round shortly. Five minutes later, when I was getting ready to go, the phone rang again. She was much worse. He was very distressed and thought she had acute appendicitis. Could I go immediately?

I went immediately, driving to their village as quickly as I could. The mother showed me into her daughter's bedroom, where I was just in time to deliver a premature baby. So not appendicitis after all. As I have said, a GP should avoid preconceptions, though here the term acquires unfortunate connotations.

Moving in 10 minutes from happily bottling wine to a home delivery of an unexpected, premature baby required some mental dexterity, especially as I was still young and inexperienced. Furthermore, though trained in obstetrics, I had no relevant equipment with me at all.

However, the girl's mother was remarkably sensible in looking for emergency essentials. She quickly found me some scissors from her sewing bag. The string was harder to come by at short notice, so I tied the umbilical cord with one of my shoelaces, and we wrapped the baby in a towel. (If circumstances and gender permit, all doctors should always wear shoes with laces, a belt, and – if wearing a tie – it should be on elastic to avoid strangulation by the mentally unwell. I have found all three useful tips, though thankfully not at the same time. The tie tip is offered from my experience when a psychopath tried to strangle me with my tie. No harm was done, though the tie was now impressively tight around my neck, with a knot more like that on a laced shoe. A colleague used a small screwdriver to prise it apart, the exercise taking place alarmingly close to my carotid arteries.)

By now a neighbour had arrived in the room, and I handed her the feebly flapping little bundle and asked her to follow me out to my car. Mum was to stay with her daughter as an impromptu midwife, and no doubt to have a chat about how it was possible to conceal a pregnancy, both at home and at school, right up until premature delivery. In truth, it is done surprisingly often.

Down the stairs we went, squeezing past the girl's thoroughly alarmed father. "What the hell's going on?" he shouted as I fled down the rest of the stairs, regrettably unable to resist calling out my congratulations on him becoming a grandfather. The wicked black humour of clinicians under high stress; it is a release mechanism.

I got into the car with my new colleague, who was holding the towel-clad baby. The hospital was nearly 2 miles away. An ambulance would take far too long to get to the house from the ambulance station in central Northampton, but nonetheless there would be all hell to pay if the baby died in my car. Such are the instant decisions we make; the risks we take.

Fortunately, the neighbour did as she was asked and did not confuse my addled mind by asking questions. I think it was the only time in my career that I felt justified in driving my Alfa Romeo Alfasud through a town as fast as I could, *Top Gear*-style, though without any handbrake turns. I put the headlights on, blowing the horn and gesticulating wildly at anybody who got in our way. Outside the hospital, I grabbed the baby from the neighbour and ran to the labour ward, crashing open its swing doors in my hurry. An alarmed midwife spun round and asked what on earth I was doing. I handed her the bundle. "Please put this in an incubator as quickly as possible." No dissent, no questions, instant appraisal – midwives are specialists in calm action during crises.

The neighbour and I sat in the little waiting area, catching our breath, at once superfluous. A phone rang; a midwife turned to us: "The family want to know if the baby is okay, and its mother asks is it a boy or a girl?"

We did not have a clue, and the infant was long gone to special care. Enquiries ensued, the reply came back, the news passed on: a girl, doing fine.

But the phone call reminded me I still had a patient back at the house. So, we got back in the car and returned to the village, though this time without the headlights, horn or gesticulations, and at a pace closer to legality.

On arrival, we found the girl's grandmother in the sitting room, ashen-faced and clutching her chest. The whole thing had been too much, and she appeared to be having a heart attack. I tried to reassure her, sat her down and asked the neighbour to phone for an ambulance while I went upstairs. The girl was fine, quietly resting in bed with her mother in attendance.

I went on seeing mother and child for some years, though we seldom mentioned that incident. Some things are best left unsaid, though there was a quiet understanding. Eventually, they moved away.

Any GP could tell similar stories. Sadly, and inevitably, they are not all so happy. The practice of generalist medicine is usually a subtle blend of science and art, of facts, uncertainty, and judgement. Errors are the price we pay for the benefits of human opinion, of making decisions when we lack the definitive information that would render choice unnecessary. Certainly, we should strive to reduce errors, erect safety nets against them, and change our behaviour in their light, but when humans are involved, we will never completely stop mistakes. Indeed, a case can be made for saying that stringent controls can at times be counterproductive.

There is a group of acute cases we might call the near misses, ones where no one was hurt, but useful lessons can be learnt. An example occurred one day in the mid-1970s when a mother in another outlying village phoned me in the middle of morning surgery about her son. The boy was known to have epilepsy and was now in status epilepticus,[79] a medical emergency. Usually, an epileptic convulsion stops after a few seconds or minutes, but in status epilepticus, it continues and requires urgent medical intervention. The practice staff ordered an ambulance as I dashed from the building, but having a head start, a fast car, and slightly less distance to travel, I beat it to the house.[80]

The boy was lying on the sitting room floor, unconscious and gently convulsing. Usually, an intravenous injection will stop the convulsions, so I took a phial of the new wonder drug diazepam out of my bag. Better drugs and techniques appear all the time, but diazepam was then the upcoming vogue. I filed a groove in the neck of the phial, as you did in those days, and snapped off the top.

Perhaps the glass was faulty. Perhaps I was clumsy in my rush. But in any case, the phial shattered in my fingers, spilling its contents and cutting me with a shard of glass. No matter how I rummaged around in my bag, finger dripping freely, there was no more diazepam. How ridiculous to be at an emergency so quickly, yet unable to treat the patient.

But then luck came to the aid of patient and doctor; I found a phial of phenobarbitone. Although this was no longer a first-line treatment for convulsions, the phial must have remained in my bag from before

---

[79] A dangerous condition when epileptic fits follow one another without recovery of consciousness between them.

[80] I left at once. Patients understood we had to attend emergencies. They either waited for the doctor to return, were fitted in with others (who went into overdrive on these occasions to make space), or rebooked.

the transition to diazepam, or for some forgotten other reason. I carefully opened it, injected it, and the convulsions stopped. The boy was sleeping quietly when the ambulance crew walked through the door a few minutes later.

It is possible that the ambulance would have had some diazepam, but this was before the days of paramedics who carry all necessary emergency drugs. In any event, all was well, but from that day I was obsessive about carrying at least two phials of every drug required for my bag, and usually more. I doubt many medical students or trainees who passed through our practice escaped me telling them this story at least once, to drum in the message: always have more than one phial of every drug you carry in your bag.

***

Of course, most acute care is less dramatic. But that is to miss the point, to ignore the rich subtlety and depth of generalism. For example, the management of an acute case has at least four parts. To manage the presenting condition of course, but often the greater challenge is to treat the individual who has that condition, including any relatives who may or may not be with them.

And you must always be on your guard for the chameleon, the severe pathology presenting as a minor or common symptom, and to look for other clinical opportunities, such as preventive measures, or the state and relevance of coexisting conditions.[81] While they are here about their troublesome rash, we can check if they have had their blood pressure recorded lately, or if a review of their regular medication has taken place. If not, we can do that now, or perhaps

---

[81] Memorably, one day I was examining a lady's sprained knee when I noticed a suspicious black mole on her thigh. I removed it a few days later at the surgery, and on the strength of the positive histology, within two weeks she had undergone wide excision of her malignant melanoma at the hospital. There was no spread, and she had no recurrence. I make no claim here other than to observe that avoiding delay is almost always desirable in medicine.

arrange it with somebody else later. Every consultation offers opportunities for checking preventive measures, and such interventions receive higher levels of uptake if done opportunistically than via postal invitation.

Avoid preconceptions. Just because there is a lot of flu about that should not short-circuit the proper diagnostic process, nor preclude consideration of the perhaps unspoken concerns of the patient. That is easier said than done. Daniel Kahneman's classic book on how we think makes this abundantly clear, and should be required reading for all those training to be doctors.[82]

For example, during the winter doctors are particularly busy, many cases may be upper respiratory infections, and time is short. But to blithely dismiss someone's sore throat as a virus, and of no concern, will be of little help to the patient who feels it is the first sign of leukaemia because their sister's leukaemia presented in that way, and the funeral was last week. And in any case, can we be sure it is not a chameleon? All serious illnesses must start somewhere. A wise doctor will commonly ask the patient's view of their condition, though with care for the phrasing: "What do you think is the problem" is a weak line, even if well intended. It courts the obvious reply: "Do not ask me – that is why I have come to see you."

And then there may be social exchanges. Did they enjoy their holiday in Madeira last month? You feel ashamed at their praise for your memory; you just read the discrete note made in their records when they saw you four months ago. But that sort of nicety helps the world go round.

General practice, more than any other branch of medicine, is itself an ongoing, chronic state. It requires a longitudinal, time-lapse consideration of the patient, rather than the inevitably staccato, flashbulb approach of other disciplines. Leaving the practice on the day I retired, crossing the car park for the last time to my car, I heard a

---

[82] Kahneman D (2012). *Thinking, Fast and Slow*. London, Penguin Books.

shout. It was a smiling young man wheeling his baby son towards me in a pushchair. As we chatted, he reminded me that I had delivered him all those years ago, and now he wanted to show me his son. I had known his father and mother virtually my entire career, from before they met and married, from before she developed the slowly progressive multiple sclerosis that by now confined her to a wheelchair. And I also looked after both the grandmothers well into their 80s; so, this baby was the fourth generation.

Not only is general practice holistic and longitudinal in its time frame, but – particularly in the last century – remarkably self-contained. Between 1983 and 1985, the overall referral rates to hospital clinics from my consultations were: 1983, 5.6%; 1984, 5.5%; and 1985, 5.5%. Furthermore, at that time we made very little use of the pathology laboratories for diagnostic investigations. We relied much more on clinical diagnostic skills than is now the case. The satisfaction gained from noting the slowed reflexes of reduced thyroid function, with the patient precariously kneeling on a chair as you tapped their Achilles tendons with a reflex hammer, or hearing the abnormal whispered pectoriloquy of a suspected lobar pneumonia, were very real thrills, especially since the latter could appear a day or two before any X-ray could confirm the diagnosis.

MEASURING WORKLOAD

From time to time, throughout my career, I recorded a consistent set of information about my workload. I describe it in the chapters on information systems, but here it offers some relevant insight into my consultations. I will take October 2000 as a typical month of my work at the turn of the century.

The split between the sexes for all my consultations was 40% males and 60% females, and with a few exceptions it was pretty consistent across the age groups.

I classified 58% of the consultations as routine, 38% as urgent, and only 4% as needing a home visit. (The reduction in home visits was one of the most profound changes that took place across the span of my career.) Only 43% involved a prescription, and just 5% a medical certificate. Referrals were fairly typical for my practice at that time.

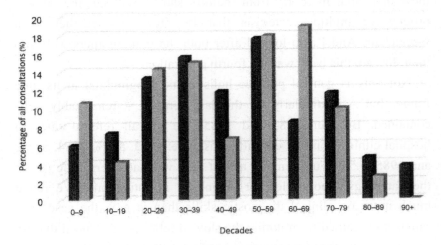

Percentage of consultations for each sex by decade.
Dark grey, females; light grey males.

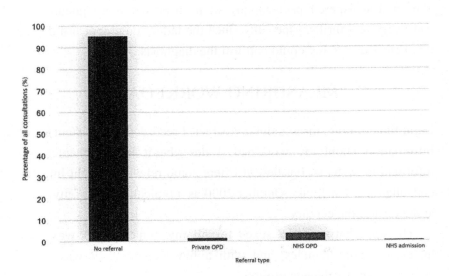

Percentage of consultations resulting in a referral elsewhere.
OPD, outpatient department.

Notice that private referrals were nearly a third of NHS ones, and in a not particularly affluent town in the Midlands. This reflected high referral rates in orthopaedics and dermatology, where early consultation with a specialist was seen as of particular importance by patients. But also notice that 95% of consultations were dealt with in the practice, without referral to specialist colleagues at all. Emergency admissions, which seem to represent 100% of most populist television series, were a mere 0.25% of my workload.

The top nine morbidity groups are also of interest. They changed in the later part of my career, particularly concerning upper respiratory tract infections – which reduced markedly – and hypertension, which disappeared completely from my workload.

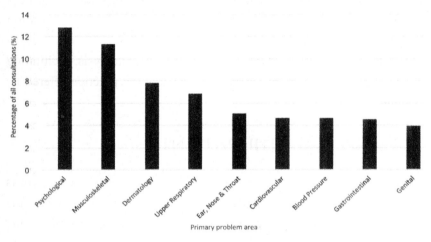

The nine most common groups of problems within my consultations, as a percentage of the total (total problem areas = 44).

I did not use the term psychological in a derogatory sense. Rather, it was to distinguish emotional and psychological problems from the psychoses – illnesses such as schizophrenia and bipolar disorder – which I categorised separately. Under psychological I included conditions such as anxiety states, mild reactive depression, relationship problems, and phobias.[83]

Also of note is the large number of patients I saw just to check their blood pressure. As I describe elsewhere, this task is more appropriately undertaken by practice nurses, and that transition was already taking place. If we assume checking blood pressures took up the same percentage of consultations for all five doctors, then in the practice as a whole the equivalent of a quarter of one doctor's time was being spent taking blood pressure, a task better performed by someone else. And it was not alone. Antenatal appointments and issuing the contraceptive pill are further examples.

Some may be surprised to see that nearly 6% of my workload involved upper respiratory tract infections. I suspect that would be a much lower figure now, following persistent health education programmes encouraging self-management.

Collecting workload data allowed that type of analysis, facilitating changes and improvements in the services that the practice offered its patients.

THE PATIENTS

I want to close this chapter by returning to the patients. Acute care is where it all begins. No matter how long you know patients, the relationships started when they came in to see you for the first time, usually about an acute condition. And long-term associations with patients – some spanning decades – are the jewels in the crown of general practice. People like John and Audrey, both of whom I had the pleasure of knowing for many years. As part of Royal Air Force Coastal Command in the Second World War, John piloted Armstrong

---

[83] It could be argued that there is a psychological element to every consultation. I would subscribe to that view, but here I only labelled a consultation in this way if I judged the primary cause of the consultation to be a significant, psychological problem.

Whitworth Whitley and Handley Page Halifax bombers on submarine patrol along the Norwegian coast, and later in the Bay of Biscay. He kindly lent me his flying log to read, a remarkable, evocative document 70 years later, which spelt out the daily life of servicemen. For example, on 17 May 1943, he not only sighted an enemy motor torpedo patrol in the Bay of Biscay, but later that day had a training session flying the four-engine Halifax with only one engine. That must have been quite an experience, particularly for his tremulous six-man crew.

John is a quietly spoken man but full of terrific stories. Apparently, as a primary school headmaster, after the war, he had to expel his own daughter from the school. (I believe she was taken back after a suitable break.) He also told me an astonishing story from his flying days. Another aircraft based at John's airfield was patrolling at 3000–4000 feet off the Norwegian coast, in winter, when it spotted and attacked an enemy ship. Unfortunately, the ship's anti-aircraft fire blew a large hole in the bottom of the aircraft.

The flight engineer went back from the cockpit to assess injuries to the crew, only to discover one man was missing, blown out of the hole by the blast.

They managed to get back to England, but as they came in to land the control tower radioed to warn the pilot that something was hanging down below the fuselage that might impede their landing. All went well, but once they had stopped, they found their missing crewman. The blast had ripped off his parachute, but part of its harness had caught on the jagged steel around the hole. He was dragged back from Norway for 2 hours, at 150 miles an hour, in freezing conditions, hanging from a bit of his harness beneath the plane. Alive, but unconscious, he was taken to the sick bay and then on to a hospital. He eventually made a full recovery and returned to active duty. John remembers him attending squadron reunions for decades after the war, albeit typically sitting rather quietly in a corner.

Getting to know people in that way is so important in family medicine. Most will not volunteer their past, but if we find it out, then that can help our clinical approach to them. Very few will have experienced the emotional toll of flying bombers throughout the Second World War, but every patient has a backstory of some kind. I trod with greater care once I knew a patient had been in Auschwitz, or the husband of another had died in a horrific industrial accident a few weeks previously.

Then there is Arthur, an engineering pattern maker and amateur model engineer. He is another quiet, unassuming man, but at the end of the 20th century Arthur was one of the greatest model engineers in the UK, if not the greatest. I have been to his house many times and seen the array of aero-engines, steam engines, and a 1:8 scale model of a 1920s racing car, but words cannot describe the intricacy and brilliance of his work. He made them all in a small garden shed, into which he crammed his few essential, carefully oiled machine tools. The model car took him six years; in every detail it runs and works just like the real thing. So, for example, the gearbox and engine worked, and water flowed through tiny tubing in the radiator.[84]

I remember his wife Joy coming to see me one afternoon. Once we had concluded the consultation, she produced from her handbag a lump of shaped, shiny metal. "What on earth is that?" I enquired.

"The engine sump; he has just finished it. Arthur thought you would like to see it!"

The car itself was eventually finished and won the gold medal and "best in show" at the model engineering exhibition that year. Years later, Arthur's enthusiasm slowly waned and eventually ceased altogether. His last model lay unfinished on the bench, which was a great sadness to him. Now well into his 80s, he simply lost the will

---

[84] Such was his reputation that a specialist motor museum lent him the parts of one of the only three full-size cars still in existence. Even that was in bits, and these lay in Arthur's garage for six years. He would take each one, scale it down to 1:8, and machine a replica.

and physical ability to press on with it. So, he shut up his cherished workshop and gave the model to me. Now the magnificent, almost-finished 18-cylinder rotary aero-engine lives in my sitting room, a marvel of model engineering.

With patients like these, there is little wonder I ran late in my consulting sessions. But this would be an incomplete description of acute care within general practice without emphasising that patients are not diseases but people. They are not illnesses that happen to be in a person, but a person who may or may not have an illness. Osler was right; we can only wholly treat a person when we know them, and when we know what makes them who they are.

GETTING THE BALANCE RIGHT

Health is a state of complete physical, mental and social well-being, and not merely the absence of disease or infirmity.

World Health Organization

Currently, there seems an almost insuperable problem in meeting all the demands put on a practice. I believe in the future we will see a more satisfactory arrangement all round, largely enabled by technology.

For now, the situation is unsatisfactory for everyone. In this chapter, I want to highlight a couple of issues that are important to patients, and then two of importance to GPs.

THINGS THAT CAN CAUSE DIFFICULTIES FOR PATIENTS

ACCESS

From the very earliest days, access has been patients' greatest problem with NHS general practice: getting to see someone and, in particular, the someone we most want to see. We can find the whole process laboured, frustrating, and annoying.

Repeatedly phoning a number that is engaged; annoying menus that lead to more irritating menus. Electronic messages assuring you, over and over again, that your call is important to whomever it is that will not answer your important call. Waiting only to find that when, at last, someone does answer, the person you want to speak to is away, or does not work on Tuesdays, or they are there but busy, or at that precise moment is apparently nowhere to be found on earth. All these things are deeply frustrating, particularly if you believe yourself to be very ill. But the ultimate inducement to blood-spitting rage is to be told that all the appointments for today have now gone. "You should have phoned earlier" incites dark thoughts when that is what you have been doing for the last 45 minutes, starting 5 minutes before the lines opened. If we could solve this one, the NHS bill for hypertension treatments would fall dramatically.

Practices will argue that things are not as bad as is often made out: early morning demand is inevitably heavy, and a patient can always be seen if there is a need. (That is another phrase practices should avoid. Of course, there is a perceived need – that is why you are phoning.)

That said, they are correct. The situation reflects the unstable economic balance I describe elsewhere in this book. Unconstrained demand exceeds available resources. Even in 1999, we were logging over 600 attempts to get through to us within the first 2 hours on Monday mornings. Of course, that was not 600 different people; it was a much smaller number having to phone over and over again because they could not get through. We only had four receptionists on duty, and that was more than in many practices. Two were available to answer the phone while the others were helping patients at the reception desk. We were doing our best, but we could not service the demand. Nonetheless, from patients' perspective the service was dreadful.

How do you meet accelerating demand with finite resources? The answer must be to employ ways that are different from those that have failed in the past. Fortunately, the cavalry is coming, and it is wearing silicon armour. Information technology is providing solutions that are already benefiting patients and practices alike. Using the WWW to book consultations at the practice or request a callback telephone appointment, are two examples already in widespread use. Video consultations can now be conducted using Skype, or similar software and apps, without actual physical contact, and at much greater convenience for the patient.

And that is the point. In contrast to the past, much of the time we do not need to go to the practice at all. A useful axiom is that a physical consultation is only required where the clinician needs to touch the patient. It is certainly not an absolute, there will be plenty of exceptions, but it bears consideration.[85] There are still those alive who can well remember how the telephone meant they no longer had to go to the doctor for absolutely everything. Perhaps they could just speak to him, and get his advice that way. But at the time no doubt some were horrified at this change in working practice.

Videoconferencing has been a part of industry for years; it is time it played a much larger role in medicine, and for the same reasons: convenience, economy, and efficiency. It can save everyone time and make much lighter use of resources such as buildings, staff, and car parks.

Secure networks such as VSee permit encrypted, live audio and video consulting between locations anywhere with an Internet connection. Recently, I have seen it used by a patient to consult experts face-to-face on two continents other than their own, yes continents, both on the same day. Sometimes it takes an extreme example like that to illustrate the broad potential of an idea closer to home. And in the context of this discussion, closer to home is exactly the point. The patient referred to was in her home for both consultations.

Naturally, many consultations would be entirely unsuited to such techniques or other forthcoming technologies, such as virtual reality imaging, but I suspect even a majority of current workload would. The

---

[85] The chance finding of a malignant melanoma described in the previous chapter offers an excellent example of the benefits of a physical consultation. No one solution is perfect; all have costs and benefits.

potential to alter and improve clinical practice is staggering, and the systems are already available if we can access them.

There is another aspect to time, and that concerns the length of each consultation. It is interesting to compare a typical 10-minute consultation with a GP with that for a complementary therapist, or a specialist seeing a patient privately. In both these cases, while the patient may well have 30 minutes or even longer, the circumstances are very different. In some ways, I would have loved to offer such appointments. Some patients would even have benefited from them, particularly those presenting with several completely different problems at the same time, a situation with which specialists seldom have to contend. GPs must bite their lips when patients enthusiastically tell them how the other day their marvellous complementary therapist gave them a whole hour for the consultation. I had to content myself by musing over their ironic choice of verb.

The GP contract covers several thousand patients, all of whom are entitled to a service of appropriate, on-demand acute care throughout the day and night. Thankfully, they never all wanted it at the same time, though occasionally it felt that way. It was simply impractical to extend the duration of consultations beyond 10 minutes when I was conducting 150 a week at the surgery, and 20 more within the patients' homes.[86] The ever-increasing managerial and administrative load consumed the rest of a long day.[87]

None of this is to dismiss the issue of accessibility. It is only to recognise the difficulties inherent in the system.

---

[86] Broadly speaking, home visits took two or three times the duration of a consultation at the practice.

[87] Occasionally, in the first, inquisitive years of my career, I mapped the time slots required for different tasks in my week: consulting, coffee break, home visits, lunch, and so on. Looking back, I had no allocation at all for paperwork or administration. Later it was quite different. That is a measure of the change that took place during the span of my career, and for current GPs the administrative load is even more extreme.

CONTINUITY OF CARE

Continuity is another increasing problem for patients. It reflects several things: the distribution of the traditional functions of the GP's work among a multidisciplinary team; changes in our society itself; and the changing career structures of all clinicians, and GPs in particular. More and more are working part-time in their practices, while pursuing other elements of a portfolio career elsewhere. For patients, this means it is increasingly difficult to see the clinician they would most like to see, let alone at a time that suits them.

One perverse consequence of the government's aim in 2015–2016 for practices to work a 7-day week could be that while that may improve patients' access to a clinician, it further reduces their chances of seeing a particular one. One way or another, general practice is increasingly aping hospitals' A & E departments. It is losing qualities that made it unique and cherished. A key example is the long-term continuity of care with a personal doctor.

So here is a problematic watershed with a conflict between the two primary frustrations experienced by patients. We can picture a seesaw with continuity of care on one end and ready access on the other. Achieving its optimal balance is, I believe, not for politicians and national, one-size-fits-all dictates. Individual practices and their patient populations should decide themselves.

But there are further complexities. With chronic conditions in particular, the very place where a long-term relationship is beneficial, the family doctor may no longer be the best clinician to do the work, and using doctors for tasks better done by nurses distracts them from the clinical work that only they can do. The detail of continuity must shift. Now it may be more important for the patient to see a particular nurse practitioner about their chronic conditions than for them to see their usual GP concerning an acute problem.

Computer records ameliorate some of the disadvantages of broken continuity, but not all. They provide an unfamiliar clinician with ready access to our medical history and treatment as well as a narrative of recent consultations. But there is a difference. Obviously, it is good that the screen in front of the stranger you consult shows your current treatments, that you are allergic to penicillin, and suffer from diabetes. But that is far from the whole of general practice. You do not know this doctor, and they do not know you. You might as well be in the A & E department. The care you receive may be technically satisfactory, but emotionally it will not be the same as it would have been with the doctor you have been going to for 15 years because you trust them, have shared deep confidences with them, and sense they know more about you than you do yourself. You feel better just for seeing them, much as patients said they did with Dr Roe. They are the "doctor, counsellor, and friend" that my partner Michael Woolmore always advocated as the role of a GP.

***

This disintegration of personal care from a single clinician gathered pace from the 1990s, when the scope of general practice broadened nationally from acute care to encompass preventive medicine and chronic disease management. Commonly, neither of these new areas of clinical practice requires a doctor; indeed, most of that work is better conducted by nurses, as discussed in the next chapter. And another phenomenon occurred. Doctors increasingly found things to do outside the practice: clinical sessions in hospital outpatient clinics, fundholding, working in the local commissioning groups, or perhaps industrial medicine.

And so the bubble burst. A breach opened in the total commitment to the practice prevalent in the 1970s; the norm of a unique relationship between patient and doctor. If the concept of personal, primary care is to mean anything, then the tensions between ready access, professional career structures, efficient use of resources, and continuity of care need to be addressed and balanced. And the outcome must be satisfactory for both patients and clinicians alike.

THINGS THAT CAN CAUSE DIFFICULTIES FOR DOCTORS

LISTS

An average of 10 minutes per consultation is usually pretty comfortable for experienced GPs, provided they are dealing with a single problem. Of course, longer would be nice, and more in line with any other advisory profession. Trickier can be the multiple consultations brought about by patients' lists of problems, or the boy brought in unannounced to be seen at the same time as his sisters, mum being confident they all have the same condition.

What is wrong with that; it seems so sensible.

And it may be. The problem is that doctors cannot assume the whole family has the same thing. They have a duty of equal care to every patient presenting to them. Common sense plays a part in diagnosis and treatment, and if two have a throat infection, chances are the third does as well. But common sense also suggests that dealing with three patients will take longer than one, whatever the problem.

As the years of my career rolled by, more and more patients came with a series of apparently unrelated issues, whether overt or covert, the expectation being that I would address them all. And the lists got longer. They could throw new GPs into a tailspin of inadequacy and frustration. By the time I retired, someone could well come in with a list of six or more problems. The reason for booking the appointment might be to review their recent heart attack, but last night a leg became swollen. "It hurts when I walk on it. It must be all the sitting around." A glance while he talks, one trouser leg stretched tight by the oedematous calf looks ominously like a deep venous thrombosis, a significant problem in its own right.

But there is more to come; his ulcerative colitis has flared up since the coronary. You remember he has had nasty flare-ups in the past, a couple requiring admission.

"Oh, I nearly forgot. My wife asks if she could go on the sick so that she can look after me."

Now, assuming greeting the patient and identifying the list took 2 minutes, we now have just 2 minutes left for each of these significant problems, of which two involve the cardiovascular system, one the gastrointestinal system, and another floats amidst medical ethics, social services, and the law of the land. That list is extreme, but most GPs would agree it is not wholly unlikely. They deal with less dramatic ones every day. Their unique combination of pragmatism, efficiency, and multitasking clinical ability does indeed justify their rather odd description of being specialists in generalism.

The lists presented in varied ways; some ill-defined, others written down like a shopping list. I quickly learnt to welcome them. It is true that occasionally their need was apparently my fault: a smiling "It is so difficult getting an appointment with you. Now I am here I have quite a list!" But usually, patients were just sorry to be placing so many issues on the table. They were surely just sensible to lay out the meeting's agenda.

If I knew there was a list, I encouraged the patient to give me the whole thing, perhaps on their original scrap of paper or I would jot it down as they ran through it. That was the point. We needed the whole list before doing anything else. Then we could plan what we could do now and what would have to wait for another time.

It was so much better than the old drip feed. Unaware of a list, you would deal with the problem the patient presented, perhaps taking your time over the rash on her finger, beneath that lovely ring her boyfriend had given her only days before. Her problem was easy, autopilot general practice. The diagnosis was a contact allergy to an impure metal of less rarity than the boyfriend had implied, the necessary hydrocortisone cream quickly prescribed. But tact and time were still required when explaining that she really should ditch the item as, sadly, it did not suit her.

You would then look up, noting with satisfaction the clock cunningly positioned on the wall beyond the patient's shoulder. You proffered the prescription with a flourish of the hand that subliminally pointed to the door.

But then, the next problem would come out, the patient settling back into the chair with an alarming permanency. Trying hard to conceal disquiet, you refocused all your diagnostic faculties onto what was usually a far more significant problem. If there was a hidden list, the first item was commonly a mere amuse-bouche before the main course. She thinks she is pregnant, or has developed double vision and headaches, or she is having night sweats and has lost 4 kg in weight.

In truth, this chain of escalating events is potentially dangerous. The "Oh, and while I am here, doctor ..." scenario is well known to any GP, but there are serious issues involved. As soon as a patient mentions a problem, anything, you are morally, ethically, and legally committed. You have just been thrown what may be a ticking bomb. You can only catch it, and cannot then deny you are holding it. If you have spent the entire appointment languidly dealing with a simple issue, grateful for a breather, and at the end, the patient introduces a far more severe matter, you are not only stuck but in the worst position to deal with it. You are aware of the heaving waiting room, and perhaps just a little frustrated by the unfairness of the world. Now stressed and distracted, you may miss the all-important clue, or dismiss some significant symptom. You may fail to spot the chameleon.

Often the only solution is to say you should meet again as soon as possible to deal with it, and that you have not addressed it in any way now. You write that in the notes for medico-legal reasons. But that has problems too. Perhaps the new issue truly is urgent and cannot be postponed, as would be any of the examples cited earlier. Perhaps the patient is about to go on holiday, which is why she felt compelled to mention it now. Or, more likely, there are no appointments for over a week. You are right to think that the world can be unfair.

The written, agreed list was a more elegant and satisfactory way forward for everyone, provided you had it at the outset. Then you could address the pregnancy or the headaches first, and just take 30 seconds at the end to tell her to take the ring off for a bit as she is allergic to the metal, and see if putting face cream on the rash helps it settle down.

Several benefits accrued from the lists. First, it was remarkable how often it was possible to group different items on the list, just as it is with an initial stab at a shopping list. Rather than the Brownian motion of wandering the corridors of Tesco in search of items from 1 to 25, you can group them. All the vegetables, all the frozen foods, and so on, perhaps keeping the wine section as a well-deserved prize at the end.

From a random list, order can emerge. Time-saving efficiency was taking place already, and the sorting and grouping process was helpful to us both. Second, with the list clearly displayed on the desk before us, we could both get a realistic idea of the time required to cover it all. Together, we could prioritise and agree to postpone some things to another occasion. Some might even be dealt with more appropriately by someone else. Many are the dental cases I have been expected to manage in my time (perhaps dental fees played a part), and the excellent Citizens' Advice Bureau was a resource far superior to me concerning almost anything beyond medicine.

Patients were almost always very comfortable with this approach. To lay out a clear plan of campaign, if necessary over several appointments, creates clarity and manages expectations on both sides, but it all starts with patients setting and presenting an agenda.

Most importantly, this approach immediately exposes the final item on the list. Where there is a list, it is often the last one that has brought the person to a doctor. Such is human nature. Many pharmacy assistants know of the nervous young lad who wants some aftershave, then some cough sweets, then shower gel. And at last – when the previous, older lady has finally shut her wretched handbag and moved away – a packet of condoms, please.

Lists were a good thing, and I welcomed them, though single problems were very much better.

THE WWW PRINTOUT

In the early days of the Internet, the WWW printout was for many doctors another bone of contention. In part, this arose from the availability of search engines. It was a new phenomenon. The caricature is assertive patients doing their research and then coming not so much to ask your professional opinion as to test your knowledge and tell you the answer. It was an odd form of power game.

As time passed, things changed. It became a commonplace for sensible patients first to investigate their concerns, and then bring that information for discussion and opinion. This was good for several reasons. With occasional exceptions, the more patients know about their condition, the better. Examples that bear ample proof of this include hypertension, asthma, and diabetes – where the expert patient is a well-recognised example of best practice.

For me, there was another point. The patient and their printout might well raise pertinent questions I could not answer. It was a golden opportunity to switch to the search engine on my computer and look up the subject together. We could do it there and then, looking up the references they had brought along, and others besides. First, this snuffed out any concern they might have about their approach – we were now doing it together. Second, and I hope less obviously, I could check up on the subject myself. Here was a clinical win-win if ever there was one.

They seemed to find this approach open and interesting. I could also show some patients how and where to do it themselves, using the sources I knew to be accurate and helpful. The WWW became a mutual information resource. As far as I recall, I was never threatened by it, but rather saw it as an opportunity for mutual benefit and assurance. It was also a chance to play with the technology during consultations, a matter of some appeal to an ageing computer geek.

***

So, where are we now? What has changed in general practice acute care, and who has benefited from those changes? How can we assess its quality?

Without a doubt, the quality of clinical care is dramatically better than it has ever been, and not just in the treatment of croup compared to 1830. Much of this is because of better training for GPs, an expanding professional literature, and readily available, evidence-based clinical guidelines. Of course, there are new drugs, but most of these are variants of previous ones, and real pharmaceutical innovation – vital though it is – happens less often than you might think. Finally, there is increasing review of working practices and results – clinical audit – and contractual incentives that encourage practices to raise their standards.

The logistics behind the improvements have also changed in ways scarcely conceivable in the 1970s, thanks to greater use of the phone and car, and the coming of the computer, the Internet, and the WWW. All these have enabled real benefits for patients.

GPs have benefited too. Their task has moved from an all-consuming vocation to a profession that is more in tune with our time. The old contractual responsibility of each GP to provide appropriate care during every hour of the year has acceded to a corporate responsibility held by the practice as a whole, and their individual work restricted to the hours of a long working day.

But not everything is better. Time to listen, empathy, and accessibility are three characteristics of a consultation that in 1964, and again 13 years later, Ann Cartwright found to be of great importance to patients. And the increasing, externally imposed requirement for administration and management within their work is an oppressive burden that threatens the willingness of many GPs to continue.

The future goal should be to retain, indeed to enhance, Cartwright's three characteristics within logistically efficient and clinically competent general practices where clinicians enjoy working. Achieving that balance is a challenge to practices, and to the NHS as a whole.

PREVENTIVE CARE

Alone we can do so little; together we can do so much.

Helen Keller

Hospital care is where most of health expenditure goes, but therein lies a problem. If the idea in our society is to use our NHS money to buy the most health improvement possible, for the most people, then hospitals do not offer the greatest value for money. Few of us hold to such puritanical, economic altruism, but nonetheless it points to a tension running through this book, the one between the individual and a wider group, or population. It is a tension that usually we choose to ignore.

A story involving the first surgeon I worked for is interesting and snaps the issue into sharp focus. It is about equity, doing the best for everyone according to their relative need, given the available, limited, resources. I have mentioned Pip Newman before, the first consultant I worked for after qualifying. During the Second World War, he had been the orthopaedic adviser to the War Office. Apparently, some weeks before a major initiative, perhaps D-Day – I do not recall – officials phoned to ask how they should best spend the available budget for orthopaedic equipment for the battlefield. "We do not have a big budget, and want to use it sensibly for equipment that will help as many soldiers as possible. What do you suggest?"

His enquirer ran through examples of the most sophisticated orthopaedic equipment of the day: Steinmann pins, external fixation rods, and so on. Pip thought for a moment, and then confirmed: "So what you want is to help as many soldiers as possible with the limited money you have for orthopaedic equipment?"

"Yes, Yes. Of course. Absolutely. What do you suggest?"

"I suggest you buy as many walking sticks as you can afford."

It is just that simple. This true story works on so many levels. It exposes our preconceptions and rationalisations about what we mean when we talk of an equitable health service for our society, "each according to need", yet one provided using a finite budget. If that is our goal, then we are going about it in the wrong way. Most of us, most of the time, do not mean it, largely because of emotional forces.

In the chapter titled "Bringing the NHS Up To Date: 1974–2005", we saw that world authorities such as Professor Barbara Starfield in the USA found that money spent in primary care provides better health outcomes than the same amount spent in secondary (hospital) care, let alone in tertiary (super-specialist) care. So why do politicians and officials charged with deploying the NHS budget incessantly talk about hospitals, sometimes as if these were the service in its entirety? If they want value for money regarding health gain, and they profess to do so, they need to change course. They need to give public health, and social and population care a higher priority. Bill Gates knows that, as does anyone else experienced in providing healthcare to the less advantaged world, where the economics of such care is seen to matter, and where the focus must be primarily on prevention, and the care of populations. They would agree with Pip Newman, and use their scarce resources for buying – not walking sticks – but mosquito nets, education and vaccines rather than ICUs. To them, the alternative would be absurd.

This chapter is about the practice of prevention medicine, of placing one stitch early to save nine later. Much of it is concerned with helping individuals as a population. The worldwide eradication of smallpox was a triumph; others are the current endeavours against polio, malaria, and HIV, and the digging of boreholes for water in arid areas. Prevention focuses down through the herd to the individual. We are immunised against measles to increase our immunity, but also to reduce the chance of exposure to the disease for everyone. It is simultaneously an individual and collective exercise. To exclude our children from a national immunisation programme is ultimately a selfish act; it relies on the actions of others to protect them.

Sometimes, primacy goes to the herd, and sometimes to the individual. Measures to detect early cancers, to check for raised blood pressure, or to use mosquito nets all have a more personal perspective than immunisation, but all are parts of preventive medicine.

Three broad groups classify the subject. Primary prevention involves preventing illness before it even exists, for example, through immunisation programmes and the use of mosquito nets. Secondary prevention means detecting an existing illness very early, before it has symptoms and when it is treatable, for example, screening for cancers or raised blood pressure. Tertiary prevention means controlling existing illnesses to try to prevent them getting worse and developing complications, for example, the management of diabetes or rheumatoid arthritis. Tertiary prevention is a subject on its own and as such dealt with in the next chapter.

Preventive medicine is in some ways best seen as a component of public health – improving the health of the population rather than just treating the diseases of individuals. In his 1988 report, *Public Health in England*, Sir Donald Acheson[88] defined public health in the following terms:

> *[Public health is] the art and science of preventing disease, prolonging life and promoting health through the organized efforts of society.*

Preventive medicine lies towards the society end of the self–society spectrum. That is the conundrum for health policy planners: to blend

---

[88] Sir Donald Acheson, a physician and epidemiologist, was Chief Medical Officer between 1983 and 1991. Acheson D (1988). *Public Health in England: the Report of the Committee of Inquiry into the Future Development to the Public Health Function.* London, HMSO.

the two inflexible, contrasting principles of competitive divisiveness and cooperative equity. In 1624, John Donne wrote: "No man is an island entire of itself; every man is a piece of the continent, a part of the main ... ."[89] So it is in preventive healthcare; we are at one time both individual and collective.

Public health is the home of the vaccination programme that eradicated smallpox from the natural world.[90] Here we also find the introduction of clean water supplies, the construction of proper drains, mosquito nets, health education, and the pasteurisation of milk. If we add societal and economic changes, such as those concerning improved nutrition, improved housing, and the output of the medical research community, we list some of the most important causes of improved health. Public health is the big hitter in improving population health and reducing health inequality, which makes government cutbacks in the public health service in 2015 all the more astonishing.

In listing contributors to improving the health of populations, we should acknowledge the research of the pharmacology industry. Antibiotics are perhaps the most obvious example of a stream of developments that have benefited millions. Others include antiretroviral drugs for those with HIV/AIDS, synthetic insulins, oral contraceptives, drugs for raised blood pressure and arthritis, inhaled steroids for patients with asthma, statins, and the remarkable aspirin. It is impossible to consider modern medicine without the therapeutic tools provided by the research laboratories of pharmaceutical companies.

And there is the research conducted elsewhere, in academic centres and clinical laboratories. One of the most profound was the work of Richard Doll and Austin Bradford Hill, who in 1951 began a study of

---

[89] *Devotions Upon Emergent Occasions and Seuerall Steps in My Sicknes.* Meditation XVII.
[90] Smallpox is extinct in the natural world, but a few secure laboratories hold samples for research purposes.

34 349 UK male doctors, the previous year having been the first to report a clear relationship between smoking and lung cancer.[91] Their study found that approximately "half of all regular smokers will eventually be killed by their habit." It reported about every 10 years after that, including the relationship between smoking and coronary thrombosis, and chronic bronchitis.[92]

Of course, politicians have played a key role in UK population healthcare. Inevitably it was governments that introduced the National Insurance Act 1911, and the NHS in 1946. It was governments that commissioned enquiries which produced influential documents such as the Dawson and Acheson Reports. And politicians are not always the vote seekers so lambasted by the press; they may well act against the grain of reactive public opinion. Which of us who is old enough to recollect, did not first object to the new law insisting we wore a car seat belt? And which of us annoyed by speed limits doubts, if we are honest with ourselves, that driving fast makes serious injury from an accident more likely?

Then there is that quiet, underpublicised and underfunded workforce of volunteers, aids, and helpers. Their commitment and goodwill are crucial, yet all too often taken for granted. They too are doing preventive work, and policymakers would do well to correct their lack of support, for the service depends on the goodwill of these people.

***

The purpose of considering all these factors is to illustrate the complexity of providing a national health service, to highlight the disparate parties involved, and to suggest that we take most of them

---

[91] Doll R, Hill AB (1950). Smoking and carcinoma of the lung. Preliminary report. *Br Med J*, 2(4682): 739–748.
[92] Doll R, Hill AB (1956). Lung cancer and other causes of death in relation to smoking. A second report on the mortality of British doctors. *Br Med J*, 2(5001): 1071–1081.

for granted. It makes our individual health worlds within an economically privileged society seem miniscule.

We are invited to go to our practice for a blood pressure check, perhaps a blood sugar test, or a cancer screen. That is passive; it is easy. Someone else does the test; the result is positive or negative; someone advises us what to do. But elsewhere, things are less straightforward. We are in charge; we are baffled by conflicting arguments between experts and not so experts about immunisation. Should we have our children immunised or not? We try to make sensible, informed decisions using streams of information that contradict each other. For years, red wine is good for you. Go ahead, have some; the evidence is clear – a glass a day helps prevent heart disease. Then suddenly, in 2016, the scientific evidence is flipped, like a pancake in the pan. The other way up now and after all they burnt the first side. Dire warnings are issued by the same scientific community that before was so sure. Now any amount of alcohol is a bad idea, but like other dangerous pastimes, such as crossing the road, done in moderation and with due care, a little is an acceptable risk. But only a little.

Most preventable deaths in the UK relate to smoking or obesity, with alcohol rising fast. There are no tests necessary for any of these; we know if we smoke, are overweight, or drink too much. The management of these is down to us, and overall many of us are not too successful at it. I know I am not. I may not smoke, but I am overweight and, according to the latest guidelines, I drink too much. Under the previous set, I was doing fine, even smugly encouraged by expert evidence that the Shiraz was fending off the Grim Reaper. Now I feel guilty and self-destructive as I slink towards the bottle.

Health promotion, the encouragement of beneficial behavioural change, is an important part of preventive medicine; at least it is where a lifestyle choice is an available option. Research in 1999 showed that GPs were keen to give health promotion advice during consultations, that many of them already did so, and that patients were interested in receiving it.[93] However, the research also showed the same doctors doubted the benefits of such advice. Of course, doctors acting as health educators regarding alcohol start at a disadvantage. There is that unfortunate definition of an alcoholic as being someone who drinks more than their doctor.

That said, GP intervention of brief advice about smoking, accompanied by an explanatory leaflet and follow-up, has long been known to be a cost-effective mechanism for helping people stop smoking and remain so after a year.[94] Here doctors have a better record. Collectively they were the first to respond to the theoretical link between smoking and lung cancer, and their subsequent reduced rate of that disease was among the first substantial confirmatory evidence of the relationship.[95]

That will always be the rub with health promotion; others can only do so much for our lifestyles. We cannot delegate the task of becoming non-smokers, of eating less sugar, taking more exercise, or drinking less alcohol. That responsibility lies with us. All others can do is ensure that we have convenient access to appropriate information and encouragement.

So, preventive medicine is partly about the individual, and partly about the population within which that person resides. Health promotion helps us improve our health and prospects. To shamelessly distort one of John Kennedy's best-known quotations, in the developed world, preventive medicine is not just about what others

[93] McAvoy BR, Kaner EF, Lock CA, et al. (1999). Our Healthier Nation: are general practitioners willing and able to deliver? A survey of attitudes to and involvement in health promotion and lifestyle counselling. *Br J Gen Pract*, 49(440): 187–190.
[94] Russell MA, Wilson C, Taylor C, et al. (1979). Effect of general practitioners' advice against smoking. *Br Med J*, 2(6184): 231–235.
[95] Doll R, Peto R, Boreham J, et al. (2004). Mortality in relation to smoking: 50 years' observations on male British doctors. *BMJ*, 328(7455): 1519.

can do for us, but about what we can do for others, as well as ourselves.

***

We should stretch the subject of prevention further, into the significant area of iatrogenic illness, conditions resulting from medical practice itself. The use of penicillin in a patient known to be allergic to it is clear-cut, as is the MRSA[96] infection contracted in hospital or psychoses induced by antimalarial drugs. Less obvious are the emotional sequelae of medical actions. But the following story illustrates how these can be of equal or even greater importance.

In the 1970s, I got to know a lovely man who regularly came to see me for a heart check-up. A minor heart attack some years previously was the start of things, to be followed by another more recently, and he was now terrified of having a third. His was not the understandable fear anyone would have in that position. It was abject, lifestyle-shattering panic. He was crippled by his fear of the third heart attack, convinced it would be fatal.

He seemed to find our chats helpful. I reassured him his heart sounded fine. "Excellent, ticking along nicely. Like a Rolls-Royce." Direct eye-to-eye contact, reassurance, positive tone; that sort of thing.

In truth, from a physical point of view, it was all meaningless. I am certain there are those that consider this dreadful witchcraft, a misuse of my position. I should have told him there was nothing I could do. At that time, preventive interventions such as modern medications, stents, and bypass surgery were not mainstream. They would argue that if he was going to have another heart attack, then that was his fate, and I should advise him accordingly.

But I disagree, and I am sure he would too if now he could comment. Indeed, there was little I could do but echo the practice of

---

[96] Methicillin-resistant *Staphylococcus aureus* is the best-known of the antibiotic-resistant bacteria.

my Victorian and Edwardian predecessors William Barr and Robert Bradley Roe. I could flourish my stethoscope like a magic wand and dispense the drug doctor.[97] It helped for a bit when nothing else at that time would do so. The stethoscope and I were there to support him, at least for a paltry 10 minutes every two or three weeks, and hopefully, he felt better for a day or two, perhaps more. Other than that, he knew he could phone me, and from time to time he did. But for the rest he had to fend for himself, to seek other props to lean on. We both knew that.

And why was he in this emotional state, the one that crippled him for the rest of his life? Because of a single, well-intentioned but misguided remark from a doctor trying to help him. After his first attack, he remained in the hospital for two weeks' rest, the clinical practice of the day. His coronary had rattled him – he was of a mildly anxious disposition – and no doubt that showed to those looking after him. One morning a junior hospital doctor tried to reassure him: "You will be all right", he breezed. "This is your first. It is only after your second you want to get really worried!"

And sure enough, after his second heart attack, he remembered this sage advice and did exactly what the doctor had ordered. He worried for the rest of his life. He worried right up until his third heart attack, in his car on the way to a meeting of our patient support group (PSG), of which he was the secretary. He died at the wheel, at the Nene Valley Way roundabout, a quarter of a mile from the practice and a few hundred metres from the A & E department.

In any case, the advice was wrong; people who have had two heart attacks may never have another, and it certainly does not help to think a third is your fate. Decades later, he would now have investigations

---

[97] The drug doctor is a term that recognises that often doctors are themselves a therapeutic agent. "I feel better as soon as I see her" is a very simple example. As I described in earlier chapters, Victorian and Edwardian doctors were masters of its use, not least because they had few other therapeutic weapons.

and procedures to prevent further attacks. But then – for him – a simple, ill-thought-out comment destroyed much of his happiness throughout the last years of his life.

***

This chapter has tried to illustrate the importance of preventive medicine, how it is much more than cervical cytology, blood pressure checks, and measles immunisation. Its value extends right across our society, indeed across the world.

PREVENTIVE MEDICINE IN PRACTICE

*The only way to keep your health is to eat what you don't want,
drink what you don't like and do what you'd rather not.*

Mark Twain

In 1973, our efforts at preventive care were the province of a part-time
health visitor attached to our practice from the local authority. She
called in from time to time, but most of her work was within child
welfare clinics and patients' homes. Her statutory responsibilities to
the under-fives took up all her time: daily home visits from the 10th
day after delivery, supporting mothers, and childhood immunisation.
Within our practice that was it, that was our preventive medicine
endeavour, other than the option of a BCG[98] vaccination against
tuberculosis at the district chest clinic.

We had no organisational systems appropriate for preventive
medicine. In fact, we had no organisational systems at all, apart from
our Lloyd-Hamel appointment book. We could not even identify our
list of registered patients, other than to wistfully gaze at the thousands
of slim, medical records tightly packed onto yards of shelves.
Incredibly, the national contract for GPs explicitly excluded
preventive medicine, with only a very small list of exceptions for
which an item of service fee was payable. Being self-employed we
could, of course, do anything we wanted, but our NHS contract said

---

[98] Bacillus Calmette–Guérin. An antituberculosis vaccine developed by
French bacteriologists Albert Calmette and Camille Guérin, remains the
standard vaccination against tuberculosis in the UK and elsewhere.

preventive work was not our job; we were not paid and had to meet any related costs ourselves.

In contrast, at the end of my career in 2006, our structured preventive medicine programme spanned the generations, from pre-conception right across to old age. It was a component of our work that was assessed externally as a part of our income assessment. Our computer systems effortlessly identified almost any subset of our patients: they showed us which interventions were relevant, when they were last undertaken, who we had contacted and when, who had missed out, who had a result in a given range, and when specific procedures were next due. We farmed our patient population regarding preventive care, the desired crop being 8500 healthy patients. Of course, no patient had to comply with the advice given, though over time the achievement of national targets inevitably increased the level of coercion practices applied to their patients. But we presented them with what the NHS considered appropriate opportunities, and we could act according to their individual response.

There were now two full-time health visitors and their assistant, until about 2004 all based in an office within the practice. That said, they were still employed externally, and the work predominantly remained their statutory duties to the under-fives. But now we employed a team of five practice nurses, and a substantial proportion of their activity involved undertaking all our adult preventive procedures.

Regarding premises, the health visitors still attended the community children's developmental clinics, but increasingly they were transferring that work to our building. The ground floor of our purpose-built medical centre contained a suite of five rooms for the nurses, to be used, among other things, for child health and preventive medicine clinics.

All this represented a dramatic development over 33 years regarding personnel, systems, and premises.

***

Back in the 1970s, we were beginning to recognise the potential for preventive medicine and needed to equip the practice with the necessary facilities. The first step, in 1976, was to establish a list of things that were worth doing. Screening was the new big thing nationally and offered by pioneering commercial operations such as BUPA,[99] which had recently opened its first screening centre in London. Who better, then, to ask for advice, particularly when it transpired I went to medical school with their research director.

Two things struck me during our discussion. First, the breadth of our programme would inevitably extend beyond theirs at both ends of the age spectrum. They were primarily concerned with working adults; we would be offering a service from infancy to old age, for everyone. So, welcome though it was, their expert advice would necessarily be confined to that for relatively fit adults.

The second observation was more surprising, that there were few interventions proven to be of value and applicable to us. I think the list just strayed off the fingers of one hand, but not by much. I do not include things patients know themselves, such as their weight and smoking habit.

But there were things we could do for adults. We could measure blood pressure, check urine for sugar, blood, and protein, perform cervical screening, and check for breast lumps.[100] On the other hand, there were things not worth doing, such as routinely checking for low thyroid function and anaemia. While the paucity of this list was surprising, it was also pleasing. It would be easier to set up than we had thought. We already catered for the under-fives; there seemed little else of merit for children and teenagers other than rubella

---

[99] British United Provident Association, a private health insurance organisation.
[100] Screening for breast cancer using manual examination provides unreliable results and is no longer standard practice.

vaccination, and we had a few useful things to offer adults. At that early stage, our thoughts did not extend to interventions for older patients, though those were to come a few years later.

Most preventive procedures aim at groups defined by age, sex, or both. Our first task was to set up an age-sex register using the system available from the RCGP. It was a simple, manual system that made it easy to identify such populations, and with secretarial assistance and a new, practice-employed nurse we had all we needed to provide coordinated preventive care, such as a well woman clinic.

A mainframe computer at the Oxford RHA held the official childhood immunisation register. Unfortunately, our updates to it, and the reports from it, were transferred on paper and sent to us by post. Turnaround could be measured in weeks. The whole thing was so slow and inaccurate that we preferred using the practice's age-sex register for our own immunisation records and the organisation of developmental assessment clinics.

Our simple preventive programme spanned primary and secondary preventive care, as well as health promotion. It worked, but was very labour-intensive. By 1981, the new microcomputers appeared to offer simplification of this and other aspects of our practice administration, but it would be several years before that prospect became reality.

***

Effective preventive medicine is mostly invisible, which is a problem. We do not see the successes. We do not see the women without terminal cervical cancer because they regularly attended for screening, and had the relevant changes successfully treated at a harmless, preclinical stage. We do not see the child whose routine chickenpox immunisation prevented their time on intensive care with life-threatening encephalitis. And we do not see that 50-year-old man whose brain haemorrhage never occurred because his raised blood pressure was noted and treated following a routine well man check-up.

Of course, we do not. But preventive programmes might receive higher uptakes if we could, if random people we passed in the street had a notice around their neck saying "I am alive because I had X, Y, or Z at my general practice".

No such thing is possible – there is no way of knowing who could wear the signs. But it might make a good television advertisement for preventive care. Just the idea emphasises how difficult it is to be aware of an intangible benefit. It is a difficulty which threatens the uptake of preventive medicine procedures, and the all-important "herd" benefits of public health policies. If immunisation levels fall below certain levels, then the benefits plummet; an example of Aristotle's "the whole is more than the sum of its parts".

In the past, such threats to the population have been well recognised by planners and policymakers. As we have seen, those setting up Northampton's Royal Victoria Dispensary in 1845 decided to provide immunisation at no charge, and in 1920 Lord Dawson, while advocating a mixed economy of payment methods for a national health service, nonetheless promoted free preventive medicine for all.

Unfortunately, the converse is not true. People are very quick to point out perceived disadvantages of preventive procedures, even if the accusation lacks sound research support. Just as we cannot identify the individual beneficiary of preventive procedures, we find few things more frightening than an invisible, lurking menace, as Steven Spielberg demonstrated in his 1975 film *Jaws*. Just remembering the pulsating, alternating chord sequence is enough to raise the pulse.

Adverse publicity focused on a perception of personal risk has had profound effects on carefully constructed public health programmes. Pressure groups formed by understandably aggrieved people are responsible for some of this, as is shallow, populist journalism. Notable here was the biased drive against the combined measles, mumps, and rubella programme. Ironically, a wish to protect our own by avoiding their immunisation increases the risk to the whole community, a community that includes our own.

The task of policymakers and practitioners is to ensure that, where they advocate an intervention, the chance of overall benefit outweighs the risks. Some elements of the media take a perverse and irresponsible pleasure in promoting stories about where things have gone wrong. And, undeniably, they do go wrong. Any beneficial intervention also carries risks, just as does driving a car, going swimming, or walking down a flight of stairs. But we do these because the benefits outweigh the risks. The pet shop is on the other side of the busy street, and we want some cat food. Or, at least, the cat does. So, we cross. The subtle balance of benefits and costs is always difficult to explain, but its inclusion in media items would be helpful, responsible, and fair. Then, of course, that would also spoil a good story.

An inherent part of preventive programmes is their assessment. It is one thing to provide a service of, say, screening for a presymptomatic cancer of some sort, but something else again to know whether your effort is having any effect, or an effect commensurate with the cost of the exercise, given the inevitable opportunity costs elsewhere. How many people are having the test, what percentage of positives are you getting, and of those, how many remain after repeat testing? What benefits accrue from a positive result, and so on. Before computers, that assessment was harder to make than offering the service in the first place. Early efforts commonly reflected more amateur enthusiasm and curiosity than sustainable, scientific rigour.

In 1976, I wanted to check the blood pressure of all the adult patients consulting me, to see if I could uncover any new cases of hypertension. I also wanted to have a look at my known hypertensive patients to see how my treatment was getting on. So, I combined the two. Later, such enquiries would be dressed up and called a clinical audit, but I was merely curious.

There was nothing fancy here. I simply listed on A5 filing cards all the patients I saw, with columns ruled for their name, age, and sex, their blood pressure, whether I already knew they were hypertensive, their smoking habit, and their weight. I also recorded if females were on the contraceptive pill because that could affect blood pressure. I still have those cards – an amusing aide-memoire of a different time.

First, I used the results to assess the management of the patients I already knew to be hypertensive. The most charitable assessment of my management would be to say it showed room for improvement, even judged by the lax therapeutic standards of that time. The best that could be said was that the study goaded me to do better. It was quite a moment – the first objective assessment of my work ever done.

The blood pressure exercise was more successful as an example of opportunistic screening, performing a screening test during consultations that were primarily about something else. A third of those I screened this way had a single diastolic reading over 90 mmHg. Of course, by no means all of those would go on to a confirmed diagnosis of hypertension, as many would have lower subsequent readings, but for sure some would require treatment. Even now, looking back at the cards four decades later, I recognise nine people who needed continuing hypertensive therapy, and there may have been more.

The prize catch of that study, if I may classify him that way, was a large, 46-year-old West Indian, who was never far from laughter. The cards show his screening blood pressure was 200/125 mmHg – high by any standards. Neither he nor anyone else knew he had hypertension, and together we treated it until he left the practice 25 years later. Perhaps he was one who could have worn a sign around his neck.

That little exercise about blood pressure was a good example of organised curiosity.[101] It was not formal research, it was not for anyone else, it was not smart, and it was not because someone felt I should do it. The term organised curiosity just reflects someone being curious about what they are doing, just as when cooking a risotto we will occasionally test the bite of the rice, to see how it is getting on.

***

By 1986, our preventive programme was computerised. Within consultations, we checked patients' blood pressure, their smoking habits, and other criteria, initially to their surprise, and entered the results directly into consulting room terminals. We used the computer to produce call letters for patients who had not been seen, and recall letters for those overdue.

That October, we sent out our first postal invitations for flu vaccinations to patients we knew to be at particular risk. The computer spewed out 250 letters, less than 3% of the list and a modest total by later standards, but a start. Now, a practice might expect to provide six or more times that number. I have no record of how many took up our unsolicited invitation, but I know some did.

These ventures into proactive preventive medicine were stimulating, but during 1987 we became aware of a potential trap. On paper, our preventive programme looked pretty good, but was it good in reality? We had agreed objectives, nurses and doctors were doing opportunistic screening during consultations, and we were running a well woman clinic, well man check-ups, and the child development clinic. One of our internal reports stated that there was "a uniform enthusiasm for preventive medicine throughout the practice". But it also noted the trap: "Our service looks good, but we may not be doing what we think because no one measures performance and outcomes."

---

[101] The term "organised curiosity" was first used by Dr TS Eimerl, one of the pioneers of research within the CGP.

We knew our programme was taking a lot of our time and effort, but could not prove it had much effect. It would be a few years before we developed adequate systems to get on top of that one.

***

A different approach, an adjunct, was to provide a system for patients to check their health status. The idea offered several attractions. First, our staff were not required very much; they could get on with other things. Patients worked through an on-screen computer questionnaire and received a printed report of results and relevant recommendations. It was a bit like a computerised survey screen from BUPA. But ours was free, and any of our patients could use it as often as they liked.

Second, patients answer questions generated by a computer more honestly than when addressing a human being, particularly about alcohol consumption. There is not much point in trying to deceive a machine about that, though a breathalyser may offer an exception to that observation. Third, and this is the backbone of health promotion, it kept the patient in charge. Finally, the report was the product of a computer. In the main, we believe computers. Spoken advice from your doctor can be rationalised ("How dare he lecture me; I bet he drinks like a fish, and I know for a fact he smokes"), or just quietly forgotten before you get home. But here was a personal report, produced in black and white by your fair hand, and even with your name and address printed in bold at the top. Here was a statement to take home and ponder over a beer, fish and chips, and perhaps a relaxing cigarette.

Our first effort was using a free system my GP brother had written a couple of years beforehand. James designed and wrote "Health Screen" to run on the Amstrad PCW, the cheapest computer he could find to keep costs down, and to help make it widely accessible. It was very popular with his patients, and in 1990 we set it up in our surgery.

We only stopped it when we moved premises in 1992, by which time 600 of our patients had sat before its modified keyboard and funny green screen, patiently answering its questions and then reading their personalised report.

James has a thought-provoking anecdote concerning one of his patients and Health Screen. She came to see him the next day in a state of considerable agitation. "It says I am overweight", she indignantly exclaimed.

"Well, with respect, I have been telling you that for some years", he replied.

"Yes, I know that, but the computer says so."

Following our move, my son Mark created a new system. "Check-Up!" was the subject of his computer science university dissertation. Ten years after Health Screen, it had the benefit of more modern technology, such as a touchscreen and a more powerful computer, but in essence, the two systems sought to do the same thing. Both were free and popular with patients, and both produced a printed report for them to take away. A survey found that 98% of Check-Up! users found it gave helpful advice and was easy to use. It helped our patients, and Mark got a distinction.

The two systems shared an important feature; they were entirely anonymous. When the patient had finished and printed out their report, the computer deleted their results. But before doing so, both systems asked if the patient would like any relevant results transferred to their medical record. Almost all chose to do so, but it was an important principle. The check-up was theirs, for their benefit and use, and they should decide what to do with the results.

**

Included in the 1990 GP contract was the requirement for practices to offer patients aged 75 years and over a home visit to assess their general health. As this was part of our self-employed contract, we did not see it an appropriate task for already busy, health authority-employed district nurses attached to the practice. We employed Margaret, an excellent ex-district nurse with additional experience in health promotion as our domiciliary nursing sister. Her role was to undertake the assessments, which in our case covered issues of physical health, emotional well-being, and social circumstances. Of over 700 letters sent out, 55% accepted her invitation, 10% declined, and 35% did not respond, even though we had enclosed a stamped addressed envelope, an explanatory letter from Margaret, and a very simple slip of paper on which to indicate their preference. Maybe they steamed the stamp to use for something else.

There were definite positive results, if modest ones, and as far as we could tell no disadvantages to patients at all. Subsequent referrals to the GP included 4% with significantly raised blood pressure (diastolic more than 110 mmHg) and 5% with sugar in their urine and a subsequent increased fasting blood sugar. Other referrals included 11% to occupational therapy for aids to daily living, 12% to chiropody services, and 4% to a social services day centre.

Those numbers may seem small, but in any screening programme, a positive return of 4% for important tests would be seen as rich pickings. Certainly, the patients liked it and uptake increased over the few years we repeated it. Eventually, sadly, we had to abandon the assessment-at-home service to free up practice-employed nursing time for work within the practice building. Resource constraints incur opportunity costs, and this service was a casualty of that equation.

The patients missed their annual check. It serves as a useful memo to policymakers: avoid raising public expectations above sustainable levels. At the time of writing, the aim is a fully functioning NHS working 7 days a week. The signs are that policymakers have once again failed to think through the economic realities of their admirable intention.

***

At the turn of the millennium, our preventive programme had matured. We were employing a full team of five nurses that spent much of its time on prevention. We had excellent computer and administrative support, well-structured policies, management protocols, audits of the process if not outcomes, and a population of patients accustomed to being offered, and receiving, assorted checks at different times for a variety of things. Also, we had the practice's range of guidelines on healthy living printed as pamphlets available in the surgery, and as downloads on our website. We wrote these ourselves, so they had the advantage of specificity compared to standard ones. For example, we could include the names of appropriate staff to contact, with direct phone numbers, and precise advice about how and when to get help.

We based our adult preventive medicine programme on the current evidence of benefit. It included blood pressure checks, tetanus immunisation, prostate assessments, cholesterol assessments, mammography, safe sex advice, blood sugar checks, cervical smears, pre-pregnancy advice, smoking cessation assistance, contraception advice, and travel immunisations. Also, we reminded patients of the value of obtaining regular eye checks from an optician, regular dental checks, and the widespread value of the community pharmacist.

Full-time administrative and computer staff coordinated and monitored the whole programme, calling and recalling patients, and conducting proactive follow-up of abnormal results with the practice's clinical team. What had started as a small acorn of an idea in 1976 had grown over 24 years into a broad-branched oak tree.

Like similar practices, we were rather proud of our system. It was evidence-based, more comprehensive and coordinated than any in the private sector, and of course entirely free to our 10 000 patients.

***

But nothing stands still for long. The thrust of centralist management gathered pace and in 2002 the government issued its set of National Service Frameworks (NSFs). Together, these showed how the government wanted to structure and coordinate the service, diminish health inequalities, and micromanage service provision within local communities. The ghosts of the *Grey* and *Red Books* floated above them as interested, if aged, spectators. *Health Improvement and Prevention: a Practical Aid to Implementation in Primary Care* was one of them, and set out five key aims and standards for preventive medicine: (1) reduce the prevalence of coronary risk factors in the population, including smoking; (2) promote mental health for all; (3) reduce the risk of cancer through reducing smoking and promoting a healthier diet; (4) reduce the risk of developing type 2 diabetes; and (5) improve the health of older people through increased physical activity, improved diet and nutrition, immunisation against influenza, and the prevention of falls and strokes.

Within all five areas, there was a focus on reducing health inequalities within the community, emphasising the population basis for preventive medicine and equity within the NHS. Our preventive programme did not have to change much at all, but it felt different. It was no longer our own invention, something of which we could be proud. We were now being managed.

CHRONIC DISEASE MANAGEMENT

Chronic disease management is tertiary preventive medicine. It is the task of managing existing, ongoing conditions to prevent their deterioration or the development of complications. In organisational and clinical terms it is distinct from primary and secondary prevention and is usually considered a separate entity, which is how we deal with it here.

Virtually every condition that continues for years, perhaps for the rest of our life, runs a course that we can monitor. When we take a long car journey, we keep an eye on our speed and adjust it as necessary according to changing circumstances. We know our destination and have a plan to get there. We monitor our fuel level and turn off the road to fill up when needed. If the oil level is low, we top it up to avoid damage to the car. It is the same with a condition such as hypertension or epilepsy.

We monitor appropriate parameters of the situation to ensure that all is as expected. Should the results suggest an undesirable change, then we can act to counter it, in so doing reducing the chance or severity of complications. If the blood pressure of a patient with hypertension rises or falls outside acceptable limits, the medication is adjusted to bring the pressure back into line. A patient with asthma may not be aware that their condition is deteriorating unless they monitor it with simple tests. By so doing they can abort an acute attack before it becomes symptomatic.

Even from these simple examples, it follows that the review of chronic conditions is well suited to exception-reporting management algorithms. If all is as it should be, we can carry on without change. But if condition A happens, do X; if the results of test B are getting worse, do Z. In our analogous car journey, the management algorithm is the satnav. You are here, so take the next left turn in 200 yards. OK, you missed that one. If possible, perform a U-turn.

Nurses are far better than doctors at following instructions. They excel at implementing structured pathways. Even when I was training in the early 1970s, research showed nurses recorded blood pressure more consistently and accurately than doctors. The skills of GPs are different. They are trained to think and behave more loosely, to use discretion and judgement in assessing multiple information streams simultaneously. They may bend the rules of an algorithm, or rationalise an abnormal result to be just good enough in this particular case. Such fluidity may not suit good chronic disease management.

Algorithms can be used by patients to manage their condition. The pathways will indicate objective circumstances in which to consult someone with additional skills and knowledge. So, if home care is not working, the patient or carer turns to the practice. If that is not working, the practice consults a hospital, and if care at the local hospital is not succeeding, then the clinicians there refer to a tertiary centre. Such stepwise pathways are inherently safe and make the best use of available resources.

One might ask why we do not just consult a tertiary care expert and miss all the other steps?

There are several reasons. Expertise is relative to circumstance. A cardiac surgeon may lack the knowledge and skills required to understand and help an individual within their everyday home life. In medicine, just as elsewhere, we need the right horse for a particular course. Another reason is one of economics. Specialist services are fewer in number and expensive, to be deployed with maximum benefit. What matters to us as patients is that we deal with a person with the appropriate skills and knowledge for a given circumstance. For the NHS, that should happen at the least cost regarding resources for the necessary standard of care. We do not use a Chinook helicopter to move a small pile of bricks. It is worth, for a moment, thinking why not?

And always there should be a tension, a rubber band, pulling us back, away from relatively scarce and expensive expertise when it is no longer needed, and back towards where we will, usually, prefer to be.

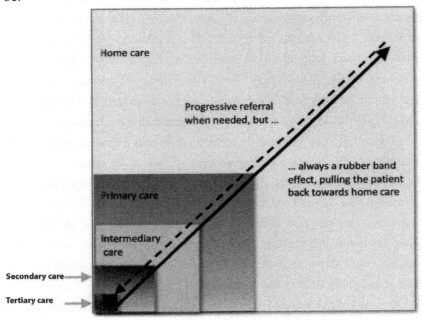

Home care

Progressive referral when needed, but …

… always a rubber band effect, pulling the patient back towards home care

Primary care

Intermediary care

Secondary care

Tertiary care

The flow and ebb of referral, although most care takes place at home or within primary care. (The areas shown are illustrative only.)

You may say this is common sense and already happens. But it does not. Every day, patients occupy hospital beds because they cannot make progress in their rehabilitation. Some call them "bed blockers", but that is ignorant and unfair. They are merely unwilling subjects of organisational failure. The rubber band is unable to draw them away from a level of care they no longer require nor want. They get stuck, no matter how hard the band pulls.

What is needed is for policymakers to shift their gaze from the shiny lights and high drama and to strengthen the facilities and resources of intermediate, primary, and home care. After all, it is nearly a century since the Dawson Report called for intermediate care centres.

***

The efficient monitoring of ongoing conditions is not a new idea. The US Institute of Medicine (now the National Academy of Medicine) concluded in 2001 that:

> *Carefully designed, evidence-based care processes, supported by automated clinical information and decision support systems, offer the greatest promise of achieving the best outcomes from care for chronic conditions.*[102]

The fact that we are living longer, together with our diet, are two major reasons why chronic disease is consuming an ever-increasing percentage of healthcare resources. Almost half the adult population of the USA has at least one chronic medical condition, and about half of those have more than one. Yet, even after its recent advances, which are themselves now under threat, the USA still has rudimentary population healthcare compared to, for example, countries in Northern Europe.

But it has many exceptions to that generalisation. When, in 2002, I visited Kaiser Permanente, a health maintenance organisation mentioned elsewhere in this book, it was running what seemed to be an exemplary system of chronic disease management. Its Population Health Management Program had a sinister sounding title, but a much better strapline: "Improving the health of a population, one patient at a time".

---

[102] Institute of Medicine (US) Committee on Quality of Health Care in America (2001). *Crossing the Quality Chasm: a New Health System for the 21st Century*. Washington DC, National Academies Press.

It focused on five characteristics: (1) evidence-based guidelines and protocols; (2) patients being empowered to look after their care as much as they felt able; (3) multimedia health education programmes; (4) the coordinated involvement of nurses; and (5) making full use of health educators and pharmacists in patient management. Underpinning the programme were integrated information systems for individual patient care, evidence-based support, monitoring the relevant population, and clinical audit.[103] I found the coordinated, rigorous, and patient-centric approach very impressive. Yes, there are differences between the NHS and Kaiser Permanente; for example, Kaiser Permanente only has 9 million registered members. And it is certainly not without its critics, but those five principles form a useful blueprint for chronic disease management anywhere.

While that is a particularly cohesive model, applied to several million patients, similar exercises have been developed in the UK. These include the publication of the DoH report *Supporting People with Long Term Conditions* in 2005,[104] which was spearheaded by David Colin-Thomé, at that time the National Clinical Director for Primary Care. The document contains a succinct model that stratifies patients into groups of relative risk, optimising the use of resources, providing appropriate care for each patient, and facilitating patients' involvement in their own care. This inherently sensible model makes best use of available resources to provide an equitable service: treating people according to their relative need within a defined population.

Like the NSF for preventive care mentioned in the previous chapter, the government published its NSF for chronic disease management in August 2002. Again, it placed much of the

---

[103] Clinical (or medical) audit is a quality improvement cycle whereby specific performance standards are agreed, mechanisms for their achievement are designed, then outcomes are assessed and changes are made to improve future results against previous performances.

[104] Department of Health (2005). *Supporting People with Long Term Conditions*. London, DoH.

responsibility within primary care, and particularly within general practice and community pharmacy. But it also pointed to the patients themselves and highlighted the importance of helping them develop into their own therapists:

> *On average, a diabetic spends around three hours per year with a health professional. This means that the patient is left to manage his/her own condition for the other 8757 hours of the year. These figures graphically illustrate why helping patients with chronic disease to understand and take responsibility for their condition is so important ...*[105]

Exactly. The first task for doctors helping with long-term conditions is to appreciate that they can usefully provide information and medication and occasionally perform technical procedures, but that the individual bears the main weight of managing the condition. My patient with the fear of another heart attack would testify to that.

Government thinking had been along these lines for several years before the publication of the NSFs. In 1999, it set up an Expert Patients Task Force to develop self-management initiatives, and the eponymous 2002 NSF incorporated its findings.[106] One of its most fundamental observations was that there is a set of generic needs relevant to most of the 17.5 million adults in the UK living with at least one chronic disease. Many of those for a patient with A will overlap B, or C, or D. They included:

> *Knowing how to recognise and act upon symptoms, dealing with acute attacks or exacerbations of the disease, making the best use of medicines and treatments, accessing social and other services, dealing with fatigue, managing work and*

---

[105] Department of Health (2002). *Chronic Disease Management and Self-care*. London, DoH, p. 1.
[106] Department of Health (2001). *The Expert Patient: a New Approach to Chronic Disease Management for the 21st Century*. London, DoH, p. 17.

developing strategies to deal with the psychological
consequences of the illness.

It is evident that patients themselves quickly acquire considerable experience in managing their particular chronic condition, far more than most of their professional advisers. The idea of the task group was to harness that experience, provide expert knowledge in readily accessible forms for patients, and encourage them not only to help themselves but to help others within lay-led educational programmes. The term "expert patient" was not a new idea. It had been in use over the previous two decades in the USA; other groups in the UK were developing the concept, and it was mentioned in the government's 1999 White Paper *Saving Lives: Our Healthier Nation.*

Now, such a shift in management from professional to patient seems a glimpse of the obvious, but at the time it was a significant change, albeit one slow to develop into anything approaching its full potential. It was clearly visible within the 2011 NHS reforms, with their central focus on the wishes and needs of the individual patient.

Research has shown many benefits for patients from the expert patient approach, including an improvement in the doctor–patient relationship, with greater understanding, mutual respect, and enthusiasm to work together, each contributing their expertise. What it does not show, at least according to research published in 2007, is a reduction in the use of NHS resources or hospital admissions.[107] Some see this as a weakness in the approach, but I would be surprised if it were otherwise. My experience has always been that the more patients (and doctors) know about a condition the more resources they wish to use in its management. Doctors find all sorts of uses for a new technology, such as the gastroscope, which facilitated a dramatic expansion of hospital gastroenterology departments. Innovation may

---

[107] Griffiths C, Foster G, Ramsay J, et al. (2007). How effective are expert patient (lay led) education programmes for chronic disease? *BMJ*, 334(7606): 1254–1256.

result in an exponential rise in costs. Similarly, as patients become expert and learn about available resources appropriate to their needs, we should consider it a plus if they use them. Better, more effective care usually comes at a cost.

Doctors have clinical knowledge of diagnosis, the natural history of the condition, its treatment alternatives, and the implications that affect choices. They also hold the key to prescribing or referral to further treatments, advice, and investigations. On the other hand, patients are best placed to build on their experience of the illness, their personal circumstances, and their individual preferences. So, by working together, patients and clinicians can better construct an appropriate, individual management plan, and then evaluate and adjust it in the light of experience and the changing clinical picture.

As I have said earlier, patients with a chronic condition require information, and here is another example where the WWW is revolutionising medical management. One of the greatest difficulties is to know which to use of the many online resources. We could point patients to ones we recommended, for example, the online library of the National Institute for Health and Care Excellence (NICE),[108] which in its own words, "is a library and information service for the NHS, available 24 hours a day, seven days a week". It offers patients "more opportunity to act as equal partners in directing their own health care through access to authoritative, up-to-date information".

Many other sites provide accessible, authoritative advice. Some are more general,[109] some offer the evidence base for therapeutic decisions,[110] and others are specific to particular disciplines.[111]

---

[108] NICE (2017). *Online Library.* [online] Available from: www.library.nhs.uk (accessed 9 January 2017).
[109] *Patient.* [online] Available from: http://patient.info/ (accessed 9 January 2017).
[110] *Bandolier. Evidence based thinking about health care.* [online] Available from: www.bandolier.org.uk/ (accessed 9 January 2017).
[111] *DermNet New Zealand.* [online] Available from: http://dermnetnz.org/ (accessed 9 January 2017).

This combination of a shift of emphasis within chronic disease management towards understanding that the patient is an expert of their own condition, coupled with the educational opportunities provided by the expert patient programme and electronic information sources, provides an encouraging prognosis for this branch of healthcare.

**

Back in 1973, hospitals monopolised the review of ongoing illness. Over the next 30 years, the position revolved 180 degrees, in large part due to the development of practice computer systems, the emergence of practice nurses, new contractual payments targeted at chronic disease management, and overstretched hospitals seizing the opportunity to discharge patients to meet their own targets.

That last point is particularly interesting. During the 1980s, our practice had developed the systems, and employed the staff, to manage many of our patients with long-term conditions, and we tried to pull them back from their tedious trips to medical outpatient clinics every few months. Frequently we were unsuccessful, even when the patient expressed a wish to have their care at the practice. Hospital tradition decreed that the follow-up of even such conditions as type 2 diabetes and well-controlled hypertension should take place in outpatient clinics. Surely, if appropriate facilities were available in the patient's practice, this was a ridiculous waste of resources.

For example, patients had to attend surgical clinics two weeks after a straightforward operation to check that the dissolvable stitches were out. I pointed out that our nurses could look at a stitch line as well as anyone in the hospital. They could even, say it softly, take stitches out.

But then in the 1990s the tide changed. Hospitals became answerable for meeting targets concerning delays for outpatient appointments. They needed to streamline their services. Suddenly general practice was, after all, the obvious place for the follow-up of such cases, and patients were discharged back from hospital clinics at a prodigious rate. It seemed that a patronising trust in the practice was no longer a prerequisite. Good things often happen for bad reasons, but they are good, nonetheless.

CHRONIC DISEASE
MANAGEMENT IN PRACTICE

When we first came to see chronic disease management as the province of general practice, we also saw difficulties. We needed a means of knowing which of our patients had the relevant conditions, when we last saw them, and when they were next due to be seen again. In the late 1970s, we did not have that information any more than having the necessary information for planned, coordinated preventive care. Computer systems did not exist, so we needed a manual disease register to identify the patients, a follow-up register to tell us who had defaulted from follow-up, and a repeat medication register to ease the repetitive task of repeat prescriptions for patients and staff alike. And we needed the clinical time to undertake the additional work.

And so, the gradual process of clinical delegation began. We have already noted that nurses are better than doctors at the algorithmic work patterns of preventive care and chronic disease management. We have also seen how a shift has taken place over the years towards patients looking after appropriate parts of their treatment. That rubber band, pulling the patient back towards their home and self-care, is as relevant in primary and community care as it is for hospitals. Some activities I undertook in the 1970s were now delegated to practice-employed nurses. And patients with conditions such as hypertension, diabetes, and asthma could be shown how to manage aspects of their conditions themselves.

My best source of information about workload was the paper-based consultation analysis system I have detailed in a later chapter titled "Information Systems: the Paper Years". It was a simple method of recording information about what I did. So, for example, August 1976 brought the end of the long, hot summer that year. It was an interesting month because it was not only near the beginning of my career but – to the month – exactly 30 years before I retired. Of my work, 2.1% involved the routine follow-up of raised blood pressure, while antenatal appointments took up 6.8%, and prescribing oral contraception 6.9%. Surprisingly, only 0.2% involved asthma (almost certainly because it was underdiagnosed at that time), but 1.8% involved the management of obesity, and 1.2% involved seeing sales people from pharmaceutical companies.[112] Finally, 3.6% included cases I termed allergy/endocrine/nutrition. In total, that came to 22.6% of my workload or 145 consultations in that month. If we assume my partners' workload was roughly the same as mine, then together that represents the best part of a doctor's entire workload being spent doing things done better, and at less cost, by others.

It took time to build up our disease register by case finding. Even in 1986, it recognised only 5.3% of our list as patients with hypertension, and 1.4% as patients with diabetes, both figures far below the expected levels. In 1998, those two were still only 9.8% and 2.5% respectively, at which time 8.8% of patients were on the asthma register. Eventually, our manual disease and follow-up register showed that about a quarter of all our patients (about 2200) required careful monitoring of at least one long-term condition.

During the 1990s, both practice and patients had an increasing interest in individuals taking a greater part in their management, echoing the societal changes described earlier. They could use devices such as glucometers for diabetes, peak flow meters and nebulisers for asthma, and accurate electronic blood pressure machines.

Patient involvement transformed the management of raised blood pressure. Previously, treatment was based on single readings, often

---

[112] That I was seeing more drug reps than patients with some key conditions shook me. I changed my policy and never again in my career saw drug company reps during consulting sessions.

taken just twice a year in a busy hospital clinic. Now that could be done after a whole series of readings, averaged for morning and evening, taken as often as patient and doctor liked, and in a more typical environment of the patient's home. We bought some electronic blood pressure machines with money kindly collected by the patients group and lent them to people to measure a series of recordings at home. As prices fell, it became possible for many patients to buy their own.

Patients now came for review of their asthma, diabetes, or hypertension already armed with data needed for discussion; their chart of peak flow rates, their blood sugar levels (later to be augmented by a glycated haemoglobin (HbA_{1c}) result taken a few days earlier), or a week of morning and evening blood pressure readings. They saw our trained, specialist nurse practitioners, who used the practice's written protocols and computer systems to manage the patient's condition.

Now a phone call from a concerned patient with diabetes or asthma could include not just the subjective "I feel sweaty and giddy, doctor", or "My breathings got bad again", but also objective information. "My blood sugar is down to 2.1" or "My peak flow rate has fallen to 200 from its usual level of over 500, and the management plan says to call the practice if it falls to 50% of average."

The availability of such hard data was a huge advance. Even a doctor who did not know the patient had an immediate objective picture of the situation. Patient and practice were working together, each contributing to the discussion of what to do next.

There are several reasons why general practice is a better place to manage chronic conditions than outpatient clinics. As we have seen, patients may have several comorbidities. Because of the very nature of specialism, patients may have to attend different clinics, on different occasions, for their different conditions. Their circumstance is less patient-focused medicine than inconvenient inefficiency.

If the management of those with less severe or complicated conditions takes place in the community, it protects hospital outpatient clinics for patients who need specialist supervision.

***

The vast majority of patients with chronic conditions require repeat medication, commonly for life, which presents an opportunity to make things easier for them. The chapter titled "Information Systems: the Early Digital Years" describes how we developed sequential, postdated repeat prescription systems, and how this also meant we could tailor our prescribing to patients' follow-up, giving additional benefit. Patient and doctor could decide when they should next meet for routine review, and then we could issue the right number of postdated prescriptions to last until that time. A significant minority of patients had to pay prescription charges, and a longer duration for each could save them money. If the medication was very costly, it seemed prudent to restrict the duration of each to two or three months, in case tablets were lost. If it was cheap, we could make the duration of prescriptions three or even six months. Our system generated gasps from some others within the NHS until we pointed out that the contraceptive pill, arguably a chronic treatment, was routinely issued everywhere in single prescriptions lasting six months.

Imagine, for a moment, that a woman taking the oral contraceptive pill had to contact their doctor or clinic every month to request a repeat prescription, then collect it and take it to the chemist for supply. It is an absurd idea and rightly never happened. But then, why should patients on repeat medication for asthma, or raised blood pressure, be treated differently, especially since, unlike the patient taking the exempt pill, many had to pay a prescription charge for every item, and might be taking the treatment for life? Common sense accompanied the advent of the contraceptive pill but, shamefully, was never applied to every other long-term medication.

Patients should insist on a more convenient repeat medication service. Fortunately, systems run by practices and pharmacies using the Electronic Prescription Service are at last coming to their aid. But it has been an unnecessarily long road.

We had first-hand experience of such systems in 2001 as a lead practice in one of the three national pilot projects to transfer prescriptions electronically to the pharmacy for dispensing, and then on to the central NHS Prescription Pricing Authority. The project is described in the chapter titled "At the Cutting Edge" and provided the ultimate in convenience. Six hundred of our patients used it with enthusiasm as well as several thousand more across the country. Sadly, the notorious and eventually withdrawn NHS National Programme for IT stopped the pilot, despite its success, and it was not until 2014 that the NHS acquired anything matching its overall excellence.

***

So far in this and the preceding chapter, I have mapped changes taking place concerning preventive medicine and the management of chronic conditions. The potential for general practice to undertake the care of populations, as well as individuals, was beginning to be used within a significant number of practices.

But not all. Ministers and the NHS faced the problem of finding ways to spread these new approaches, and so help reduce the inequalities of service provision that the government rightly held as one of its principal aims. What was required was a method of persuading more practices to undertake primary and secondary prevention, and chronic disease management, and to do so to a set of national standards.

Governments had toyed with the external management of general practice before, notably in the 1990 contract, but never to the extent now seen as necessary. The independent contractor status of GPs remained an obstacle. The profession's negotiators insisted, as would any other body, that additional work should receive additional remuneration. Some outside the profession argued that these activities were already included in the GP contract to provide "all necessary care" for patients. However, that apparently reasonable, enticing gambit was countered by the precedent set in the late 1970s and 1980s. Here the government was hoisted by its own petard. You will remember that early GP contracts had explicitly excluded preventive medicine, and governments had agreed on additional payments for a small number of "items of service" such as night calls, immunisation, maternity services, and contraceptive services. Similarly, hospitals had long monopolised chronic disease management, at times actively blocking its repatriation to general practice.

Few could seriously deny now that coordinated programmes of preventive medicine and chronic disease management were new, additional work for most practices.

The outcome was the introduction of the controversial QOF. It is controversial mainly because of the manner of its negotiation as part of the new contract introduced on April Fools' Day 2004. The QOF set practices' targets founded on sound evidence of benefit to patients. Given the semiautonomous, self-employed contractor status of GPs, it was a skilful arrangement. Achievement of the targets was optional rather than compulsory, but the accompanying income made the scheme attractive to practices, as of course was the government's intention.

Initially, the QOF had four main areas within the work of a practice: (1) clinical; (2) organisational; (3) patient care experience; and (4) additional services such as screening and maternity services. Each area had its set of targets, and practices scored points according to their level of achievement against each one. The more points you achieved, the higher your target-related income.

The government hailed the negotiated contract as a triumph, but what happened next caught politicians and the DoH by surprise. The QOF ignited most GPs' latent entrepreneurial flare. They did what the scheme intended them to do, they did it well, and they did it more quickly than the DoH had expected. Within two or three years, they had achieved what the original QOF scheme assumed would take five, and consequently, their incomes rose more quickly than anticipated.[113] Inevitably, there appeared to be little short-term gain for this expense, for preventive medicine and chronic disease management are long-term strategies. However, the QOF did some things quickly. It raised operational performance and produced a welcome consistency across the country. But for the press, it was the financial effects that earned the QOF and the contract notoriety. "Greedy GPs orchestrate massive pay hike." That type of thing. It was indeed large, but QOF payments were the direct result of extra work resulting from a contract negotiated by the government.

Here it gets interesting. There was now a choice of approach for politicians. Within a couple of years, a large majority of patients with chronic conditions were being monitored to consistent standards, a remarkable feat and in its speed of implementation perhaps a unique one internationally. Equally, for the first time, the NHS offered critical preventive procedures to most people in the UK. These were triumphs of population medicine. In place now were steps to reduce inequalities of provision and raise standards of care. Politicians and civil servants could take credit for introducing all of that.

Or they could adopt another approach, one that responded to a populist opinion fuelled by shallow journalism. They could criticise GPs for making too much money. And that is what they did.

One problem with assessing the clinical effect of the QOF is that,

---

[113] There were also other elements to the negotiated contract that caused consternation. A particular one was the removal of GPs' contractual responsibility to 24-hour cover for their patients.

as is usually the case with NHS initiatives, it lacked adequate piloting and assessment. Without that, it is hard to interpret the effects accurately. Very few areas of the country had sets of comparable data from before and after the introduction of the QOF. One such area was Shropshire. Dr Mary McCarthy reported statistically significant benefits there in both the organisation and clinical outcomes, in particular concerning diabetes.[114,115] So soon after the introduction of the QOF, improvements in investigation results must be taken as a proxy for clinical improvement itself, and in Dr McCarthy's studies, there was a marked improvement in investigation results following the QOF.

Dr McCarthy also pointed out the advanced state of chronic disease management within the NHS compared to other countries, citing the November 2009 report from the Commonwealth Fund,[116] which surveyed primary care physicians in 11 countries, including Canada, France, Germany, the UK and the USA. As discussed elsewhere in this book, the report is controversial in its general methodology but, that said, the UK came out top regarding chronic disease management.

The NHS infrastructure is ideal for preventive medicine and chronic disease management with its registered lists of patients covering 95% of the population. It has highly computerised general practices with specific clinical codes in use since 1992. Beyond that essential, national infrastructure, Dr McCarthy concludes that financial incentives can lead directly to improved clinical care and significant improvement across all the relevant clinical areas.

---

[114] Tahrani AA, McCarthy M, Godson J, et al. (2007). Diabetes care and the new GMS contract: the evidence for a whole county. *Br J Gen Pract*, 57(539): 483–485.

[115] Tahrani AA, McCarthy M, Godson J, et al. (2008). Impact of practice size on delivery of diabetes care before and after the Quality and Outcomes Framework implementation. *Br J Gen Pract*, 58(553): 576–579.

[116] Commonwealth Fund (2009). *Health Policy Survey of Primary Care Physicians*. New York, Commonwealth Fund.

The results from Shropshire offer a particularly clear example of the inclusive, population-based service lying at the heart of the NHS. The QOF is an initiative of which the NHS should be proud, as should the politicians and civil servants who introduced it.

***

Chronic disease management in general practice, like its preventive healthcare cousin, changed dramatically over 30 years. In the 1960s and 1970s, it began as a hobby for the curious enthusiast. It then blossomed in some practices within the early years of microcomputers, progressively taking over from hospital outpatient clinics. But the consequential inequalities of care were a political issue, and they precipitated centralised standardisation through the QOF.

The next stage, the effect on population care of introducing CCGs and local strategic plans will no doubt be watched with interest.

PART FOUR

A PRACTICE'S ORGANISATIONAL TRILOGY

As with other organisations, a practice is built on a trinity of its premises, organisational systems, and those working within it.

Unlike hospital staff, GPs may be self-employed, independent contractors to the NHS. They are responsible for every facet of the practice and its staff, and for the provision of care to the list of several thousand patients.

Part Four considers the infrastructure of a practice, both in general terms and through the prism of the development of my own practice.

A BETTER PLACE TO PRACTISE

We shape our buildings; thereafter they shape us.

Winston Churchill

The idea of building large, purpose-made buildings for general practices is not as recent as you may think. It goes back nearly 100 years, again to Lord Dawson's model, which, among other things, proposed a national primary care system with GPs working within health centres. However, despite being a highly influential doctor, president of the RCP and physician to the king, his proposal met with stiff opposition from the medical profession.[117] That said, there were landmark examples of the idea, including the 1935 purpose-built Pioneer Health Centre in Peckham, and the Finsbury Health Centre built in 1935–1938.

The idea gained greater traction later when central strategists developing the new, cohesive NHS saw health centres as a logical step. They could place under one roof their administrative staff, community nurses, and the still independent GPs. One of the first of these was the William Budd Health Centre, built by the local authority in Bristol and opened on 16 September 1952, by the Minister of Health, Iain Macleod. A year later it was reviewed in the *British Medical Journal*:[118]

---

[117] Despite his landmark report, Lord Dawson of Penn may best be remembered for administering lethal injections of morphine and cocaine to his patient, the dying King George V, supposedly to ensure the king died before midnight, so as to be reported in the morning papers, rather than less suitable later editions.

[118] Parry RH, Sluglett J, Wofinden RC (1954). The William Budd Health Centre: the first year. *Br Med J*, 1(4858): 388–392.

It is a prefabricated single-story building containing six general-practitioner suites, each with its own waiting-room, surgery, and examination-room; a main waiting-hall; a large office; a staff room; a medical treatment room; and the usual offices.

The GPs were not in partnership, and the centre merely provided their branch surgeries. The suites were to be used either by GPs or local health authority staff, but in general the former used the centre during mornings and evenings, the latter in the afternoons. This was an early example of what we now term hot-desking; little in life is truly new.

What I find most interesting in that *British Medical Journal* article is the stated purpose of the centre in 1954:

The aims of basic group practice are identical with those of ordinary general practice. The primary aim is to provide patients with the highest level of diagnostic and therapeutic service attainable outside hospital, to inconvenience the patients as little as possible, and to preserve the best elements of personal service – all at a cost the patient (or better, the community or nation) can afford.

The authors then conclude:

We think this is being achieved at the William Budd Health Centre without formal financial partnership but with the advantage that each practitioner firm maintains its individuality and that the patient can indeed be sure that he will see the doctor of his choice and not any one of half a dozen or more different members of a group practice.

The centre was to provide practitioner and local authority work to a housing estate of 30 000 people. The original staffing arrangements included a sister-in-charge, a deputy sister, and three nurses, two secretaries/typists, one general clerk, two porters, and two part-time sisters. Because of the unusual circumstances in the area, full nursing cover by day and night was provided, with the nurses living in a nearby hostel.

The William Budd Health Centre demonstrated remarkably prescient thinking and a well-focused solution to the needs of a particular community. It was well used: by the end of its first year it had 10 000 registered patients; this involved a workload of about 33 000 consultations with doctors and a further 9700 with nurses in the treatment room. (On the other hand, a cynic might observe that two-thirds of the housing estate had not registered with it even after 12 months.)

But this was only branch surgeries, not the main practice building. Its strength lay in being open 24 hours a day, with nurses always available and doctors on call. It appeared an exemplary solution to helping a community with special needs, but one too costly for widespread replication. Nonetheless, its DNA can be seen in current out of hours centres.

Developing health centres was slow, not least because of financial austerity in a post-war economy. That seems to have been the view of Dr John Hunt, the visionary London GP and joint founder of the CGP. Together with Dr Guy Ollerenshaw, a GP in Skipton, Yorkshire, he published his thoughts. Just three months after the *BMJ* review of the William Budd Health Centre they wrote:

> *While accepting health centres in principle the country, through its governments, has viewed with dismay the costs in relation to the few doctors they serve, so that their number is now strictly limited.*[119]

They came up with an alternative, cheaper solution. It would still be funded and built by the local authorities but simply be a local resource centre for primary care. While the William Budd Health Centre

---

[119] Ollerenshaw JG, Hunt JH (1954). Family medical centres; a new type of health centre. *Med World*, 80(5): 509–516.

provided branch surgery facilities for GPs, Ollerenshaw and Hunt's idea for a family medical centre would have no rooms at all for regular GP consulting. It would have diagnostic facilities, such as radiology and pathology, and a consulting suite for visiting specialists to see patients alongside their GP.

There would be local authority clinics, nursing facilities, and an operating theatre for minor procedures. It would be open to all primary care professionals to use as they wished and be a centre for communication between public health, family doctors, and staff from the local authority. In the authors' elegant words, it would "sit between the hospital and GP surgery; replacing neither but helping both."

After a stormy gestation, the Ollerenshaw and Hunt's ideas crystallised in 1956 into the Peckham Medical Centre in London. The idea was to help the 80 GPs working within 2 miles of the location by providing them with a resource centre of their own. Ollerenshaw and Hunt went on to write:

> *They will continue to work from their own surgeries, but in this centre, they will be able to meet their colleagues, ancillary workers and consultants and receive much help in the immediate diagnosis and treatment of their patients. It will also encourage them to develop close liaison with the local authority clinics.*

He saw the centre being convenient for the 33 000 patients living within three-quarters of a mile of it, reducing their journeys to and from hospitals for services done equally well locally and at less expense. It would lessen the workload of hospitals and be a place for fruitful meetings, both formal and informal, between healthcare professionals.

Despite the logic of this argument, the Peckham Medical Centre remained an exception rather than the rule. Perhaps primary and secondary care were too focused and insular to meet in the middle.

Hospitals, acquisitive by nature and distrusting of general practice, did not want to let go of anything, and general practice was all too often a very underdeveloped affair regarding structure. In 1966, the year Alf Ramsey and Bobby Moore were busy winning the football World Cup, the results of a revealing survey found that 60% of GPs were working from converted houses built before 1900, and that only 65% provided a toilet for patients, 18% an examination room, and 9% a treatment room. Creating additional, shared facilities to help primary care was neither welcome to hospitals nor a priority for most GPs.

Now, over half a century after the Peckham Medical Centre, locality diagnostic and treatment centres serving the local community may well emerge across the country, as NHS policy squeezes out more and more of the hospital sponge into the community, and with CCGs keen to keep as much within their control as possible. In the chapter titled "Building for the Future", I refer to these as intermediary care centres, arguably a kind of upgraded version of Dawson's recuperative centres, a variant of the Peckham Medical Centre, or the cottage hospitals that closed in one of the NHS "reforms" of the last century.

***

Following the 1965 Charter and 1966 contract, GPs began building medical centres using national funding arrangements such as the Cost Rent Scheme. Cost rent enabled GPs to finance the building of their premises, and the government then paid GPs rent for their use for NHS general practice. This avoided the government having to find the capital for buildings, while providing an attractive option for GPs. It was an early form of a private finance initiative. Such moves into larger, converted or purpose-built premises were further encouraged by another element of the contract that followed the Charter. Not only was money made available to help with the employment of staff, but there was also a grant for GPs who worked in group practices, and such groups required larger premises.

In 1966, the CGP published a perceptive design guide.[120] An article in the Daily Telegraph on 28 February 1967 summarised it under the breathless heading *"Leading family doctors and architects pave the way today for the transition of general practice from a cottage industry into an efficient front line service"*. It said:

> *They have produced a design guide on GP centres of the future in which groups of doctors will practice and be assisted by nurses, social workers, secretaries and receptionists. The authors believe that nurses and social workers could take over much of the work done by the GP, such as revisiting patients at home, following up attendances in the consulting room and carrying out clinical, therapeutic and diagnostic procedures.*

The proposal was for buildings different from local authority health centres, the William Budd branch surgeries, and the shared resources available at the Peckham Medical Centre. Crucially, GPs themselves would build and own them. They would be the practice's base, with other services and organisations there at the discretion and invitation of GPs.

Despite many practices building premises using the Cost Rent Scheme, health centres had not gone away. As discussed earlier, although products of the 1960s and 1970s, they were still very much in use, combining community services and primary care practitioners within one building. GPs also avoided the capital costs of owning a building – they just paid rent to their health authority landlord. Nonetheless, health centres have never attracted a majority interest within the medical profession.

And so, the main forms of primary care buildings evolved. Health centres got off to a good start and took the lead, only for GPs' own

---

[120] College of General Practitioners (1966). *Design Guide for Medical Group Practices*. London, CGP.

medical centres to overtake them. The third form, intermediary care centres, which include locality resources, will inevitably become more common in the years ahead. The ideas behind all three of these have been around for decades, but their realisation continues to reflect economic priorities and the availability of funding.

FROM A STABLE FOR HORSES TO A CENTRE FOR CARS

In 1928, our practice had a separate surgery, the one established by Drs Roe and Cooke in the stable behind No. 20 Billing Road. The building was smaller than a single garage today and probably built for a horse and trap. After conversion, it contained three cubicles and a small waiting room in the middle for patients sitting with the receptionist; the dispenser was to one side and the doctor to the other. Perhaps this basic accommodation was created by erecting partitions between the stalls.

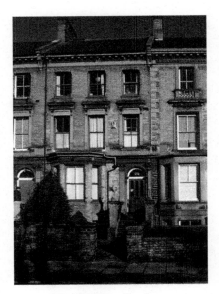

No. 20 Billing Road.

It is hard now to picture the scene. Mrs Roe hung her washing out in the waiting room, though presumably not during consulting sessions, and the little Roes' bicycles and toys were stored there also. Patients arrived and departed along the back lane behind the house, where, until the 1990s, I remember the silhouette of the converted stable as white paint on the garden wall.

The start of the NHS brought a significant logistical change. Chemists now did the dispensing, which meant our dispenser's cubicle was freed up to be a second consulting room. Now there was even room for an examination couch. Previously, all but the simplest examinations took place by special arrangement, either in the doctor's house or at the patient's home.

And that is how it was when my partner, Chris Elliott-Binns, arrived in 1955 to join Jim Mitchell. Chris remembered there were still tack hooks on the ceiling, and he shared his consulting room with the lawn mower.[121] He recalled that the thin partition walls had no sound insulation at all, so "patients who sat interminably in the waiting room could at least amuse themselves listening to whatever was going on in the two consulting rooms."

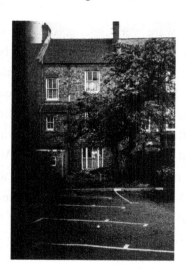

The back of No. 20 Billing Road, showing the car spaces in place of the original stable but before the modern conversion.

---

[121] Elliott-Binns C (1983). How general practice emerged from the dark ages. *Medical News*, 13 October 1983, pp. 4–8.

IN FROM THE STABLE

In 1962, the surgery was moved into the house, to more comfortable and appropriate facilities. The long-serving stable received a brief stay of execution, serving time as a garden shed before eventually being razed to make way for a tiny car park. When Michael Woolmore joined them in 1964, all three doctors had elegant consulting rooms on either the ground or first floors. With the Woolmores eventually moving out to live in Wellingborough Road, the front basement room was sublet to the Samaritans for a token fee. This benevolent arrangement ceased in the early 1970s when the new trainees, of which I was the third, required the room.

We were still using paper records, piles of which were carried back and forth around the building by receptionists clattering up and down the linoleum-covered stairs. This was hardly efficient; in any case, the steep and narrow Victorian stairs were unsatisfactory for patients, particularly if they were very young, old, or severely ill. Things changed a bit for the arrival of the fourth partner, but not much.

There was inadequate office space for the staff, and the waiting room was too small, having previously been that cosy consulting room of my first consultation a couple of years earlier. We adapted the small, first-floor bathroom as a treatment room when our first practice nurse arrived, but it was woefully inadequate. We had no common room; the building had no central heating, and there were still only four or five car parking spaces for the doctors and staff, and none at all for patients. And then, of course, there were the steps and stairs. We had to do something.

***

BACK TO THE FUTURE

We engaged Aldington and Craig, an architectural partnership with a national reputation and based near Aylesbury, and used the NHS Cost Rent Scheme to finance the project. No suitable plot for a new building was available within our practice area, but Peter Aldington designed a magnificent extension in the garden at the back of the house, a space-age steel and glass, open-plan reception area, office, and waiting room.

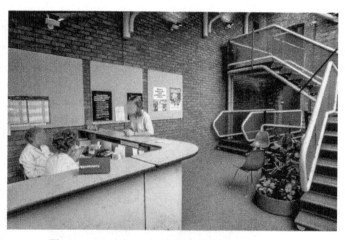

The new reception area at No. 20 Billing Road.

The angled, glazed roof soared three storeys up the back of the house, with top-quality fittings from Concorde Lighting, white-painted steel, plants everywhere, Herman Miller's Action Office furniture and Charles Eames chairs in vivid green. He removed the steep stairs within the house and, rather than concealing the new ones, made a feature of them within the extension. They were a striking structure, with white-painted steel walkways, and short flights of steps rising between small seating areas.

The reception area is the shop window of any practice, and ours was spectacular, placing us squarely among the architectural avant-garde anywhere, let alone just within general practice. The

Architectural Review was enthusiastic, commenting that the waiting area harked back to the idea of a "grand conservatory, full of light, white paint, glass and green plants."[122] Occasionally architectural students came to admire such things as its design and engineering, for example, its clever use of space, and its three-storey high, unsupported brick wall from which, nonetheless, hung the steel and glass roof!

The architect also rearranged the interior of the house. The top floor was now entirely for administrative purposes; the converted basement was the domain of the nurses, complete with a treatment room and an operating theatre for minor surgical procedures. The doctors now consulted once more on just two floors, with half of all consultations taking place on the ground floor. Far beyond our expectations, the architects had met all the main points of our daunting brief.

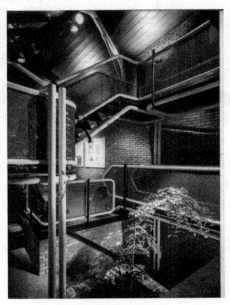

The new, avant-garde staircase at No. 20 Billing Road.
Photograph © Richard Bryant.

---

[122] *Architectural Review*, September 1983, pp. 70–74.

To me, the building was a heady triumph. It provided liberation to those working within it, considerable functional improvement for patients, and it was visually stunning. But, interestingly, none of the older patients I talked to when researching this book in 2007 had much recollection of it. One of them in passing described the reception area as "a rather strange, white bit in the middle of the building", but none of the others made any mention of it, even when gently prompted. A lot of water had flown under their different bridges in the 25 years since we left that building for new premises; nonetheless, the point should not be dismissed. After all, they remembered the original building with its gas fires, difficult stairs, and homely lighting, even though that was even earlier in their memories. Perhaps it was indeed an odd, alien experience for some, maybe many. For good or bad, at the time patients were stunned by the architecture and likened it to being in a space station.

Architecture in the 1980s could be quite brutal. Some would say it still is. Like modern abstract art, it could be beautiful and magnificent to the attuned, but strange and unfathomable to the majority. Was our extension designed for us, for the patients, or perhaps even in part for the architects themselves? It was a brilliant response to a demanding brief. It was aesthetically stunning to those with a modernist bent and remarkable even to some with other tastes. But no one could accuse it of possessing a comforting, homely feel. In contrast, the architects cleverly retained those qualities in the rest of the house, where we consulted.

Its Achilles heel was that we had not addressed the parking problem. But worse was to follow. We knew from a survey that 70% of our patients came to the surgery by car. Now the town council introduced restricted parking with residential permits in all the surrounding streets. We were on a busy road, marooned, even lacking a convenient bus stop.

In the briefing process, we had dismissed the lack of parking as being beyond our control. So, we ignored it; we ignored an elephant standing quietly beside us in the room. Similarly, we were so focused on the excitement of being able to meet our current needs, against all our expectations, that we disregarded allowing for their expansion in the future. That was not in the brief either, though the CGP's 1966 report on design referred to earlier had specifically mentioned it; if only we had read it. And then, of course, there were still the stairs – and no lift.

In the 1982 conversion, we had an architectural jewel that fitted the brief like Lycra, but we omitted two cardinal requirements: adequate parking and space to expand. By 1989, after just seven years, we had outgrown the building, and two years later admitted defeat and moved on.

A CAR PARK WITH A VILLAGE IN THE MIDDLE

My partner Allan Leroy found a plot about three-quarters of a mile to the east, on the site of a disused paint factory in King Edward Road. Better still, within the town, it was closer to most of our patients' homes than had been the case in Billing Road. As architects, we employed Bundy and Rodgers, a partnership based in Market Harborough and another experienced in designing buildings for general practice. We were keen that the new premises should embrace primary care in its broadest sense. Our initial notes for the architects offer an insight into our thinking in 1992:

> *Most obviously, primary care will integrate pharmacy and physiotherapy with general practice, but opticians, dentists, counselling and complementary medical techniques such as acupuncture will also be involved. Indeed, such people as the Community Health Council and a local councillor should be considered for inclusion in the practice's Patient Group if the*

practice is indeed to become part of the community, sensitive to local needs.

It is likely that the practice will eventually contract with a central purchasing agency to provide a raft of services to the local community, including the provision of secondary care services. The practice may or may not undertake procurement activities itself but will inevitably be involved in needs assessment exercises and the commissioning of services for its patients within the local health community.

What we really wanted was a large car park and a primary healthcare village of conventional and complementary services. This was Allan's vision, but it appealed to all of us as a means of supporting holistic primary care. However, there were only five of us, and there were real questions about whether we could afford to build such a primary healthcare paradise. In the end, we had to abandon the village idea and agree that another local practice should share a more conventional building, and the costs.

Within the Christchurch Medical Centre, our two practices were conceptually semi-detached neighbours in a two-storey building.

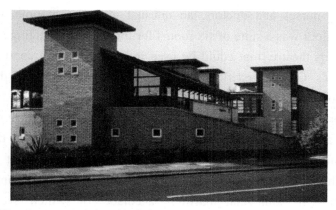

The pharmacy and dental building at the Christchurch Medical Centre.

We shared a lift, so all functions could extend over two floors without inconveniencing patients. Each practice had an outer third of the building, with its own front door, and the middle third was devoted to shared facilities, such as services, lift, health education room, staircases, and kitchen. A second building, in appearance a miniature version of the main one, housed a pharmacy and dental practice – a vestigial echo of Allan's original, primary care village.

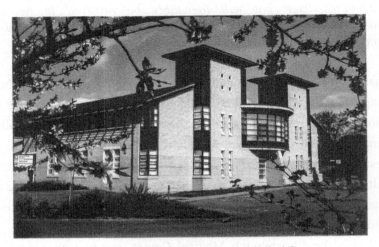

The main building of the Christchurch Medical Centre.

In our half of the building, we divided the clinical space equally between nurses and doctors, an unusual idea at that time. On the ground floor was a suite of six rooms for the nurses, including a minor operations theatre, that could be used individually or in combination for clinics. On the first floor were five consulting rooms for doctors. Both floors had a back-office area for administration.

Shortly after completion, the Christchurch Medical Centre won an annual award from the Royal Institute of British Architects as the best new building within East Anglia. It also won a Civic Trust Award from the town council for its contribution to the environment; a welcome, if somewhat baffling accolade of which we were nonetheless very proud. Our medical centre was a triumph, and the patients loved it. For one thing, they could park, and for another, it had a lift. It was the first bespoke building we had ever had, and no matter how brilliant the extension and conversion at Billing Road had been, my goodness the functional difference was enormous.

Then again, try as we might, we knew it would not last; that with the passage of time both building and car park would shrink in functional capability. This time, we had included at least some capacity for expansion, and an extension was completed in 2010, well after my retirement, giving more consulting and administrative space to both practices. But there were still echoes of our extension 25 years previously. You can often increase the size and functionality of a building, but until there is a radical alteration in the patient–practice interface, the single biggest problem for convenient practice premises remains the car.

BUILDING FOR THE FUTURE

A major issue for providing healthcare buildings concerns a tension between convenience and technical facilities. What do we, as patients, really want? How can the NHS provide us with a friendly, efficient, and convenient high-quality service from buildings fit for purpose and that use resources wisely?

The crucial point is that most patients, most of the time, want a convenient service within their community.[123] Bristol City Council realised this in 1952, building the William Budd Health Centre on an estate of 30 000 people, even though it had other practices near its perimeter.

Until 1990, when government intervention prevented this, I referred patients to any suitable hospital for their particular problem, no matter where it was. Together we balanced convenience, timeliness, and expertise. I used the local general hospital of course, but also teaching hospitals in London and Oxford, rich seams of swift opinion and almost immediate admission for patients with non-urgent conditions. Occasionally, I referred even further afield.

But in my experience, most patients did not want to travel. They wanted to stay with the hospital nearest their home in Northampton, even if they had to wait much longer for treatment. They felt it would be more convenient not only for them but also for their relatives. The lesson for economists and pro-marketeers is that geographical convenience usually matters to patients.

So, what would provide a cohesive, efficient system of medical care facilities within the NHS?

---

[123] Specialist hospital services are increasingly pooled and centralised; therefore, society is adapting to the need to travel to them, but that does not deny the desirability of geographical convenience.

The ideal would be a continuum of services across a series of related locations, both physical and within cyberspace. As a patient's need for increasingly sophisticated services increases, geographical convenience is progressively traded for the availability of that expertise. So, while a primary care practice or chemist will relate to just part of a town, a tertiary care transplant centre may serve several counties.

While accepting that no one model will suit all circumstances, we can still consider how this gradient of services might look in the future, remembering that most care takes place at home and the least in the most specialised of hospitals.

LOCAL CARE

The first level of service would be one of maximum convenience to most patients, but with the consequential lowest provision of sophisticated technical services. We are increasingly familiar with hospital-at-home facilities, but what we need even more is primary care at home. The technology is there, and we should expect to use it within medicine just as in so many other aspects of our lives. We can communicate online with our bank, supermarket, chemist, bookmaker, or airline; we are long overdue the ability to do so easily with our general practice and pharmacy. It is starting. There are already some excellent online services, and the extension of this trend will revolutionise primary care.

We already have email, mobile phone text messaging, face-to-face audiovisual communication, electronic devices that can monitor our blood pressure, heart rhythm, blood sugar, or oxygen saturation levels, and apps that remind us to take our medication or attend for a blood test. There are already authoritative information resources available online, and we will eventually access our medical records and management plans online. We will become our own expert patient, and with a suitable gadget or mobile phone we will be able to manage much of our care anywhere, either at home or even when abroad.

Such ideas cast aside the old convention that we must go to our doctor's practice for almost any form of interaction. They would align medicine with current behavioural norms and expectations; they would be convenient for everyone concerned. And with fewer patients needing to journey to the practice, there would be more space in currently overstretched car parks and waiting rooms, prolonging the useful life of some buildings.

So, our home should be the first medical building in our daily lives. On economic grounds alone, the NHS would do well to ensure it offers the best facilities possible so that we can undertake the appropriate care ourselves. I can envisage the day when going to the surgery is actually the exception rather than the rule when our activity is compared to that in the 20th century, with a profound reduction in footfall through the door.

***

When our needs exceed the possibilities at home, we require a convenient practice within our locality, with adequate public transport and parking, and containing the primary care team. Here, as now, will reside the hub of our NHS experience. It should be the home base for our electronic medical records, and our points of contact with members of the primary healthcare team (PHCT). Crucially, it should remain the access point to the NHS when we use it of our own volition. As I have said already, with two exceptions, you cannot go to hospital without an invitation. For its part, as well as dealing with our acute care needs, the practice should coordinate the use of specialist services, and the management of our preventive medicine and chronic conditions.

Why? Surely, we can go wherever we wish for medical care, provided we can gain access. Of course we can, particularly for one-off matters. But if the NHS wants to provide cohesive chronic and preventive care, then the buck has to stop somewhere. Someone must organise and run them, to invite patients for appropriate services at the right time, and ensure action follows results. A practice and its list of registered patients is historically the site for this activity. The arrangement is endorsed by government through various policies, and most recently the QOF system, and the practice list still seems the most appropriate unit of population. If we lose that coordination and accountability, it is the socially and economically disadvantaged who will most likely fall through the cracks of scheduled care. The reduction in health inequalities for which successive governments claim enthusiasm would go into reverse. Uncoordinated healthcare is dangerous.

There are of course other means of getting a clinical opinion, such as drop-in centres, pharmacies, private consultations, out of hours centres, or by the misuse of A & E departments. But these should not diminish the central coordinating role of general practice. Over 95% of the population is registered with a general practice. It is the smallest unit of population within the service, and it is from these practice widgets that a hierarchy of ever larger populations is built up, through CCGs to the entire country. Some other countries have a similar registered structure, but most do not, and of those many envy the ones that do.

So, for our second building, I believe it is in everyone's interest to ensure that general practice develops to its full potential. It should be geographically convenient for patients, operate from purpose-designed, renovated or new buildings, have well-trained staff in adequate number, and be well equipped. Importantly, such a facility can take pressure off hospitals.

***

There will be times when we need services our general practice lacks, yet ones that in themselves should not require a trip to a hospital. Examples include a chest or joint X-ray, mammography, some ultrasonography, speech therapy, and physiotherapy. A community diagnostic and treatment centre could provide these along the lines of John Hunt's Peckham Medical Centre, or those described even earlier in the Dawson Report.

Both Hunt and Dawson envisaged hospital specialists coming out into the community to see their patients. It is hard to think of an outpatient clinic that could not be moved in part or as a whole to a community setting, with benefit to patients. It is primarily because of convenience for specialists and investigation departments, and marginal though definite benefits in running costs, that outpatient clinics are within hospitals; it has little to do with satisfaction for patients.[124]

A community investigation and treatment centre would be a pragmatically sensible compromise between the economic inefficiencies of clinics taking place in individual practices, and the costs and inconvenience of maintaining them in a hospital setting. For example, the burgeoning number of patients with cancer could receive their routine, specialist follow-up in a place that geographically is more convenient to them, offering a smaller-scale, homelier atmosphere than a busy hospital clinic. Patients loved the old cottage hospitals, and planners should consider why that was so.

The centre could also be home to the community's out of hours services, again echoing the 24-hour service provided by the William Budd Health Centre and the pooled diagnostic and treatment facilities of the Peckham Medical Centre.

So here, after the home and primary care centre, we have this third building, one providing more specialised and costly services, but still

---

[124] Similarly, I make the rubber band argument elsewhere that much of the current work in a general practice could be transferred to the patient's home.

at less expense and inconvenience for patients than a hospital. I shall return to this building later, for it could have a further function.

As mentioned in the chapter titled "Bringing the NHS Up To Date: 1974–2005", authorities such as Professor Starfield have shown that it is in primary care that the maximum health benefit can be derived from a given financial investment. If the NHS wants value for money regarding health outcomes, and presumably it does, it would do well to provide first-class primary care with supporting, community-based, investigation and treatment centres.

But to be clear, it is not a question of the government taking money from hospital budgets to spend on general practice and other primary care providers. The NHS needs efficient, effective hospitals. Rather, we should draw closer to the expenditure on healthcare in other developed countries, and use some of that additional money to maximise the function of general practice and primary care. That requires a dramatic change in the understanding, attitudes, and priorities of national policymakers.

HOSPITAL CARE

Hospitals should only conduct those elements of patient management that the community cannot, or should not, provide. That is a statement of the obvious, but an obvious statement that is broadly ignored. They will remain in two forms. First, there will be local hospitals for the bulk of services, that is, those that are sufficiently frequent to be appropriately managed there. And just as primary care is a sieve for secondary care general hospitals, so these hospitals are sieves for even more specialised services, such as neurosurgery or organ transplantation, positioned within regional centres.

So, the structure of our hospitals should remain in broad outline that in existence since before the NHS. Its current disadvantage is that inadequate investment in the community resources described earlier, the first three buildings in the chain, has meant that local acute care trusts in particular have become clogged repositories for an unnecessarily broad range of services.

And that is the point. Where appropriate, acute care trusts (general hospitals) must be able to discharge patients to intermediate care centres, to be cared for at a level between home and hospital. But those intermediate care centres do not exist, so patients fit for discharge, but not yet fit for home, remain in hospital. The smooth transition from home to hospital and back becomes jammed, and the resulting back pressure bears on the second costliest point in the service – the general hospitals.

Intermediate care centres could provide care in its broadest sense, combining primary care, social services, and hospital-at-home arrangements. Here too, midwives could concentrate much of their maternity care. In at least some places, the functions of the community's investigation and treatment centre could be based there, amalgamating all the community and intermediate care facilities in one site and again echoing the ideas within the visionary Dawson Report.

Thus, there would be a progressive trade-off across a spectrum that shifts from geographical convenience, generalist familiarity and competence, economy, and a "small is beautiful" experience through to increasingly refined technical sophistication, specialist expertise, scarcity, and cost.

Happily, such a model not only provides an appropriate service for patients but is also economically sensible, transferring unnecessary work from expensive hospital facilities back into the community. We can look again at the rubber band. Conceptually, there would be a piece of rubber band attached to each of us, anchored in our home. If we needed to go to a more specialised service, then the rubber band would stretch. But when we no longer needed that level of provision, it would gently pull us back, through the intermediate layers, towards our home.

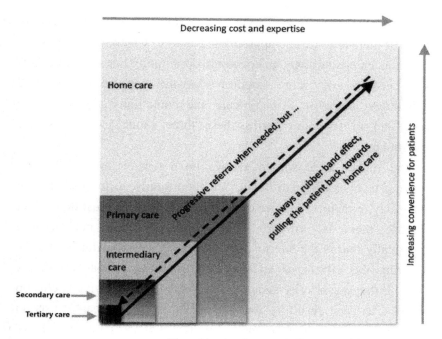

The rubber band concept of care provision.

For it is our homes where we want to be, as long as our health permits, particularly when we are old and increasingly infirm. That is the overriding message to come out of *Being Mortal: Medicine and What Matters in the End*, Atul Gawande's moving and informative exploration of the later years of life.[125] (It is a book that should be tube-fed to every medical student and doctor.) And home is also where healthcare economics wants us to be.

***

You might well say that all I have done is describe the present position. It may well seem that way, but it is not. Over the years, too much emphasis has been placed on hospitals, with a relative paucity of

---

[125] Gawande A (2015). *Being Mortal: Medicine and What Matters in the End*. London, Profile Books.

investment in community services. The rubber band principle only works if there are safe and appropriate places to which we can return.

Home care is not only an economic opportunity but something that will become ever more important as the population ages and technology improves. Primary care and community services come next, and in economic terms these three should come first for investment.

The rubber band should always be a tension on the system, drawing us ever closer to home. We should only go to hospitals, let alone stay in them, when our clinical need means we must do so. Not because there is nowhere more appropriate and not because historically that is the site of clinics or technical procedures. We are suffering the effects of an understandable but mistaken train of thought, that our priority should be hospitals to the relative exclusion of all else. The result is that hospitals, and acute care trusts in particular have become expensive storage cupboards into which we pile anything and everything. And then we complain of the clutter.

Tertiary care units are an interesting case study. They do not have the notorious bed blockers, and they do not deal with conditions that could be dealt with elsewhere. They are masters of controlling their throughput, only accepting appropriate cases and discharging them at the earliest safe opportunity. Why can they manage to do this? Because they discharge patients back to the local hospitals, the acute trusts. The rubber band works well for them; the system only dams up further downstream.

I do not pretend any of this is new. We all know it; Dawson knew it; current policymakers know it. They just do not base their strategic plans and resource allocations on it. The great mental shift, the uncomfortable change of direction, is to accept that if our society is to make the best use of available resources to provide the maximum benefit to the population, a concept enshrined in the founding principles of the NHS, then priorities must change. The current supremacy of hospitals for resources needs far more sensible balancing with those for primary and community care.

If you were establishing new health services elsewhere in the world, perhaps in poorly developed countries where resources are very limited, you would not start at the most expensive facility, where highly specialised care is provided to a few individuals, and work down to the cheapest, where far simpler methods provide effective care to much larger numbers of people at less cost. That would make no sense. You would not start by building an ICU, no matter how tragic the relevant cases may be. You would start with public health, preventive medicine, health education, aid workers, nurses, and doctors in the communities, and then work up as resources permit. That makes the best use of the money available.

But, of course, we have a problem with our emotions. We find hospital services (at least the ones we like to think about) so exciting, so needy and pressing, so televisual that they are the obvious priority for NHS funds. And when we are seriously ill, it may well be that only a hospital can help us. That seeds powerful emotions. The Nobel laureate Daniel Kahneman has written about how intuition and emotion influence our views and decision-making, and not always for the better.

Policymakers have to weigh harsh economics with public emotions, and often emotion wins. Such political pragmatism can lead to decisions that are economically unsound. For example, since the birth of the NHS, public health, preventive medicine, and health education have contributed more than hospitals to the health of the population, yet they are the poor relations when it comes to resource allocations.

***

Primary care and general practice have a long way to go regarding buildings and facilities. Even in 2008, two years after I retired, almost half of UK GPs were still working in converted houses or shops; there were few examples of diagnostic and treatment centres, and very little use of remote, online consulting. Almost all cottage hospitals had been closed for years.

I was fortunate to work in two buildings that were fit for purpose and of superb design. They made me glad to work there, to expand what we were doing for patients and ourselves. Churchill was right. Buildings that we shape ourselves do indeed allow us to do more, and so help shape what we do and do not do. His observation needs extending to a coordinated plan throughout the NHS, and as the population ages, we need it ever more quickly.

If we are to improve the performance of NHS hospitals, then surely we must reduce the stifling demand we put on them. We can do this not so much with seemingly unending further investment in them, but with greater investment elsewhere.

Here the shift of accountability and resource allocation to CCGs may hold the whip hand. They may do what governments have failed to do. We can return to my trip to Kaiser Permanente in Southern California. There, faced with fierce market competition, the efficient use of available resources mattered. No expensive doctor would do anything that someone else with the appropriate skills could do instead. Their clinical buildings within the community had specialists and generalists working side by side, and there were more than two nurses employed for every doctor. A surgeon and generalist could consult each other just by knocking on the next door; they could get to know each other over a cup of coffee. They were a team. There was much of the William Budd Health Centre about the buildings.

Similarly, hospitals were seen as necessary but expensive resources. A patient's additional day in the hospital represented wasted money. Kaiser Permanente invested in the resources to move patients away from hospitals as soon as their clinical condition allowed. The rubber band worked because they had the downstream buildings and facilities to which they could draw patients safely and appropriately. My impression was of a cohesive, coordinated organisation.

In many ways, the UK CCGs can now provide a similar structure. With demand increasingly outstripping resources, they may want to follow similar lines. Governments should find a means of helping them with the necessary capital expenditure. In the early days of computers within the NHS, innovative GPs led the way, investing their own time and money in developing systems, but it was when governments provided appropriate incentives regarding finance and staff allowances that the movement took off generally. It could be helpful for the government to enable a CCG trial of community facilities such as I have outlined. Quite apart from any other consideration, I believe it would ease the burden on local hospitals and allow them to improve their performance. But for once, let it be a proper trial, with an objective, academic assessment of costs and benefits.

No one model will suit all areas; diversity is essential. But expecting acute care hospital trusts to continue as clinical and social repositories because we have not provided more appropriate, alternative facilities is a pathway only too clearly doomed to failure. Perhaps, by 2020 we might see clear examples of the rubber band gradient across coordinated buildings from home to tertiary care. That would be an appropriate date, for it will be the centenary of the Dawson Report, which first described such a model.

INFORMATION SYSTEMS: THE PAPER YEARS

Look up at the stars, and not down at your feet. Try to make sense of what you see, and wonder about what makes the universe exist. Be curious.

Professor Stephen Hawking, London Paralympic Games 2012
Opening Ceremony

GPs require a broad spread of information, not only covering the whole spectrum of clinical practice, but also operational information to underpin programmes of preventive medicine and chronic disease management. They also need the information necessary to run the practice as a business organisation. Taken overall, this information requirement is in a different order of magnitude to any other group of clinicians.

This chapter explores the 60 years of development that have produced the technical infrastructure fundamental to modern general practice.

BEFORE 1975: THE PHASE OF PLAYFUL CURIOSITY

In the 1950s and 1960s, most objective assessments in general practice were amateur in their nature. They were like a toddler's naïve, playful curiosity, of a GP simply wanting to explore his work. "How many of my patients with diabetes are on insulin?" Simpler still: "How do I produce a list of my patients with diabetes?" Few could do that accurately.

Now we answer such questions by pressing a few buttons on a computer keyboard, but those predigital days were an information desert. Playful exploration is at one end of a spectrum of enquiry that has formal research at its other. No such activity had been encouraged within general practice until the formation of the CGP in the mid-1950s.

That initial, playful curiosity quickly turned into what Dr TS Eimerl, one of the pioneers of research within the CGP, termed "organised curiosity". Progress was rapid, driven on by unfettered entrepreneurial endeavour.[126] Different strains of registers and tools sprouted from general practice like the savannah grasses after rain. It was an exciting time for those who were so inclined, the day of the enthusiastic amateur.

Some of these individuals, who sought to push the boundaries of general practice, moved naturally into the committees and hierarchy of the evolving CGP, where mutual support further fuelled the engines of their creativity. Within such esoteric circles, their thoughts moved from the tactical (how to help themselves) to the strategic (how to extend the perceived benefits throughout the profession), so that all GPs and patients could reap the benefits. The playful, individualistic pioneers had become evangelists, and – perhaps inevitably – then moved on again, to become global enforcers.

So, here is the same progression we see in education, from the wide-eyed curiosity of the innocent toddler, through systems invented by enthusiastic teachers to help children learn, and on to the use of information for imposed formal assessment and validation. Eventually, that became a legal requirement to practise. General

---

[126] Here, I use the word entrepreneur in the sense defined by Greg Watson: "a process through which individuals identify opportunities, allocate resources, and create value." *Entrepreneurship, Education, and Ethics. Definition of Entrepreneurship* [online] Available from: http://tinyurl.com/z9toyyl (accessed 9 January 2017).

practice had moved from the nursery to school, and on to enablement through public examination.

Of course, there will always be a place and opportunity for curiosity. It should be strongly encouraged, for it is the seed corn of creativity. Its diminution in opportunity, and even in perceived importance, is a regrettable consequence of the dominance of formal structures. But the days when organised curiosity was the only show in town, with its scraps of paper, cards, and exercise books, have gone forever. Ultimately that is down to a single invention – the microcomputer. It was this that enabled the development of systems for population care within general practice, but crucially, it also allowed the enforcement of the use of such systems.

Before computers, it was impracticable for all but a few research practices to collect and store accurate data, to analyse them as routine and to use the resulting information for the betterment of their work. The time is fast approaching when no working GPs will remain who experienced the need to create paper systems themselves if they wanted to explore, to do things better, in an organised way.

Before the late 1970s, most GPs were busy enough with the individual patients who went to see them without getting involved in population care. All they needed was a theoretical knowledge of medicine and background information about the patient; they stored most of that in their heads.

Since 1911, there had been a paper medical record, but its greatest significance to the doctor was that it was the state's mechanism for determining their remuneration. Every page of the Lloyd George stationery still contains a small column within which the GP could mark an "S" or "V" for the location of each consultation. Every year, the local executive council (an administrative but non-medical body) gathered in all the records of a doctor's "panel patients" and reviewed them, by hand, to determine how many surgery consultations and home visits the doctor had undertaken. From this, they calculated the

GP's recompense for the previous year. It seems incredible now.

Apart from anything else, this annual external audit of all the written medical records was a remarkable nationwide breach of medical confidentiality. It may be charitable to suggest it is one reason why most GPs wrote little in the notes other than to mark that column. It was also the first example of NHS GPs recording information about their practice work for the use of external administrators or managers.

A disadvantage of keeping few notes was that doctors then relied heavily on their memory and intuition. One morning in my first week as a trainee at Billing Road, I sat in with Jim Mitchell. As mentioned earlier, Jim was a remarkable, traditional family doctor who seldom wrote notes at all. Commonly, he would just enter the date. This was surely a nod to his past use of that little column on the record card, where he would have entered the date and then either a V or an S, depending on whether the consultation was at the surgery or the patient's home.

In one consultation, a patient returned to report happily that his recent illness had subsided.

"Good, good," said Jim from his chair. He often repeated words like that.

"Quite better, then? All your symptoms gone?" Brief and said with an encouraging smile, an affirming nod of the head.

"Absolutely, doctor. I am fine now. I am back at work."

"Excellent. Excellent," and after a few further exchanges, the patient left the room.

"I am sorry, but I did not quite understand that case," I said. "What had been the problem?"

"I have no idea," Jim replied, and pressed the buzzer for the next patient.

That was not quite as dreadful as it may seem. Clearly, Jim knew what was wrong at the previous consultation, when it mattered. What mattered now, with no notes to refer to, was to establish if the patient was better than he was before, and apparently, he was. Jim's remarkable pragmatism may have reflected his horrific experiences in the war. Even his visiting list was succinct, and in the 1970s we could each have 4–8 visits a day. He would jot down notes in shorthand in his diary. Perhaps the odd surname or a number: "19" might be all he needed; he knew the rest of the address and the patient. But in the months before he retired, even Jim could see the problem he was about to leave us, and tried hard to write brief resumes in the notes of patients he had seen for years. And brief they were, but better than nothing.

PAPER SYSTEMS

As a trainee in the 1970s, I had time for playful curiosity. For a few months, I recorded information about every patient I saw on sheets of foolscap[127] paper on my desk. There were columns for what the problem was, the patient's name, age decade, and sex, whether they were seen in the consulting room or on a home visit, and if I admitted them to a hospital. It was a sort of daybook, and the results gave me a modest, objective insight into what I was doing. I still have those sheets, and looking at them recently I remembered at least a third of the patients listed.

After a few months, I tired of that and created a more structured system of workload analysis, using large sheets of paper liberated from the practice's accounts ledger. These were magnificent, nearly the size of today's A3[128] paper, and printed with multiple lines and columns. I allocated the rows and columns to the characteristics I had recorded in the day sheets, but with more space. I now added such things as any investigations undertaken and whether I issued a certificate.

---

[127] A size of paper measuring 330 × 200 (or 400) mm.
[128] A standard European size of paper measuring 420 × 297 mm.

APRIL 1977

			0 – 9		10 – 19		20 – 29		30 – 39		40 – 49		50 – 59		60 – 69	
			F	M	F	M	F	M	F	M	F	M	F	M	F	M
		INFECTIOUS DISEASE														
2	0	Acute D & V														
4	8	Flu-like Illness														
1	2	MALIGNANT NEOPLASM														
13	9	ALLERGY/ENDO/NUTRITION														
4	3	DISEASES OF BLOOD														
39	19	MENTAL DISORDER														
2	4	CENTRAL NERVOUS SYSTEM														
1	0	MIGRAINE														
5	1	EYE DISEASE														
12	14	EAR & NOSE DISEASE														
135	7	1st OTITIS MEDIA														
3	6	CARDIOVASCULAR SYSTEM														
6	5	HYPERTENSION														
0	3	ISCHAEMIC HEART DIS.														
7	6	RESPIRATORY SYSTEM														
1	5	ASTHMA														
1	1	CHRONIC BRONCHITIS														
24	5	ACUTE U.R.I.														
12	6	GASTROINTESTINAL SYSTEM														
1	2	Peptic Ulcers														
5	0	Gall Bladder Disease														
9	5	GENITAL SYSTEM														
32	0	Pregnancy														
2	0	URINARY SYSTEM														
1	0	1st U.T.I.														
34	10	SKIN DISEASE														
34	19	MUSCULOSKELETAL + TRAUMA														

Part of a monthly consultation analysis sheet.

There were 46 rows on each page, so I invented a classification of problems, heavily based on the major sections of the World Health Organization International Classification of Diseases.[129] I still had a few rows left, so I added some specific conditions of particular personal interest. One was otitis media, an infection of the middle ear, partly because of an impression, a hunch, that I was seeing more boys with this condition than girls and wanted to see if that was true. I put little pencil marks in the relevant cells for each consultation and added them up at the end of each month.

I was inadvertently creating a paper version of a future spreadsheet, though this was before the advent of the microcomputer. Indeed, when I began using computers, I just transferred the paper

---

[129] World Health Organization (2016). *Classifications*. [online] Available from: www.who.int/classifications/icd/en/ (accessed 9 January 2017).

system onto a spreadsheet without significantly changing the design, and let the computer do the arithmetic for me.[130] Before that, I had spent a long evening each month adding up the pencil marks in over a thousand cells on the previous month's grid and then produced totals for each column and row. The drive for this worryingly obsessive behaviour was that the process gave me unrivalled details of what I was doing. That mattered to me, and I used the ledger sheet log for well over a year before its transfer.

*** *** ***

More fundamentally, the priority for all practices was to organise the medical record envelopes. They crammed the handwritten notes and correspondence into the infamous Lloyd George folder, an A5-sized envelope designed, no doubt, to fit snugly into a capacious Edwardian pocket for home visits. (Interestingly, in the 1980s, much the same sartorial thought must have occurred to the designers of the 3.5-inch floppy disc, because it was just the right size to fit in the much smaller shirt pocket of informal Silicon Valley.) Many practices improved the notes by buying treasury tags to hold the contents in chronological order, and some designed printed summary cards to go at the front.

Our own version contained the patient's significant conditions, relevant family history, allergies, immunisation record, and dates of preventive medical procedures. We persuaded a pharmaceutical company to print them for us, as well as a yellow, follow-up record for long-term conditions.

---

[130] My analysis of 13 500 consecutive consultations revealed many things, one of which was that the two sexes had an identical incidence of otitis media. Interestingly, this is at odds with published data, which report a higher incidence in male children. So, perhaps my hunch can be seen as right according to subsequent published research, but wrong in the experience of my own work!

D.O.B.				DISEASE INDEX:						NAME:			
FOLLOW UP REGISTER:													
INITIAL INVESTIGATIONS:				HEIGHT:						PROBLEM:			
										RELEVANT PAST HISTORY:			
Date	B.P.	Wt.	Cig.	Urine	Fundi	Urea	Bl. Sugar	T4	Management			Follow Up	See Notes

Our record card for chronic disease management.

Taking a firm grip on the value of colour coding, we also used a blue card for listing repeat prescriptions. Together with the age-sex and disease registers, we had a very useful information system at modest cost. But it was fragmented and complex.

GPs flexed their ingenuity to come up with ever more sophisticated manual systems. The RCGP came to the fore by pioneering various models, including the very successful manual age-sex register. However, they were all time-consuming to use and designed primarily for research. Very few GPs tried to apply them to everyday practice.

The loose-leaf appointment diary made the greatest impact. From 1961, Lloyd-Hamel Ltd provided it free to practices, and its uptake was remarkable. In 1952, only 2% of practices used an appointment system of any kind. Even in 1963, that had only risen to 5%. After that, uptake took off: to 33% in 1967; 50% by 1971; and 70% in 1976. Nonetheless, these figures demonstrate the organisational lassitude among the body of GPs at that time. The Lloyd-Hamel appointment system was as close to a free lunch as they were likely to get, yet after 15 years, 30% had not accepted the invitation. But by 1989, the

Lloyd-Hamel system was so widely used as to be the de facto standard, omnipresent on reception desks, with its six consulting sessions ruled vertically across its width, and timed rows of appointments throughout the day. Even in 1992, a common perception was that no available computer system could match it for flexibility and ease of use, and that was probably correct. But it would be disingenuous to argue that appointment systems were primarily brought in to help patients. More than anything, they helped doctors control demand and organise their own time.

It was inevitable that GPs should seek to improve their working conditions as well as the efficiency of their practices, that is, to shift from an almost total vocational commitment to their patients to a more equitable balance. So, the simple appointment system, together with the increasing number of group practices, were the start of a movement away from the individual towards what Professor Peter Spurgeon of Warwick Medical School terms the functionalisation of general practice.

He draws a parallel with a small business being taken over by a larger one. Initially, there is an innovator, an individual, doing everything. But on being taken over, he is told he needs a head of IT, a finance director, and so on. Single-handed GPs were innovators, feeling they were sole providers of healthcare services; something they must work out how to do themselves. If they then came into a partnership, they felt in some ways taken over. Apparently, they needed someone to do the finances, someone else to run the staff, and perhaps yet someone else to manage the building. It was no longer quite the same. And even clinical tasks became functionalised, with nurses performing tasks previously done by doctors, and doctors specialising within the practice in subjects such as skin diseases or diabetes. All these things can easily be justified; on balance, they are a good thing. Nonetheless, there has been a diffusion away from the vocation of a personal doctor towards the function of general practice.

In the context of this chapter, such segmentation requires more information and therefore better information systems.

CARD-BASED SYSTEMS

In the 1970s, the college's compact, structured age-sex register was the most successful means of maintaining a convenient register of patients. Small cards measuring 12.5 cm × 7.5 cm contained the demographic details of each patient registered with the practice.

There was a separate register for each sex, one pink, one blue, each with partitions for each year of birth.[131]

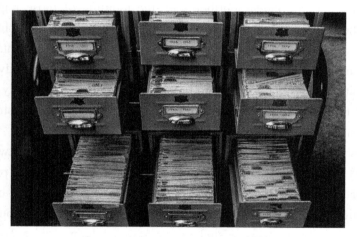

Our practice's age-sex register in 1980.

For the first time, a practice could easily identify all its patients of a particular age group and sex. For example, it could quickly find all its 40-year-old females. Maintaining this additional register in parallel to the patients' records was inaccurate, but a leap in the right direction.

---

[131] If you think you know which sex had pink cards, you are probably wrong. Pink was for males (as it had been for boys before the 1930s, denoting a paler version of what, then, was red for men). Perhaps this was a bid by the designers to buck 1970s convention, but more likely it was down to an error at the printers.

It may seem incredible that the FPC held similar card-based registers for all the patients in each practice within their jurisdiction. Maintaining those registers was a large part of their work, and they were even less accurate than those in practices. I remember the medical registration department at Northamptonshire FPC resembling a small, modern call centre, with rows of people sitting at desks in an open-plan office, manually entering and editing registration cards. In 1981, research found that the patient's address was incorrect on 8% of age-sex register records in practices, but an astonishing 17% of those at the FPC. Bear in mind that the FPC was responsible for maintaining lists of patients registered with each doctor so that they could pay practices appropriately. Furthermore, the totalling of those registers was how the NHS purported to know how many patients it had in every district and region in the country! It is a staggering thought.

This inaccuracy is hardly surprising. There was little incentive for patients to report a change of address to their doctor and virtually none at all to tell the FPC, even though the back of their NHS registration card stated this requirement.

Patients who moved home could easily be registered with two (or more) practices at the same time. Each practice would be paid a capitation fee for looking after the patient by FPCs unaware of the situation, and giving rise to GPs having "ghost patients". It could be difficult to know they existed (or perhaps no longer existed), their notes lurking silently among the rows of 10 000 others. Occasionally, you chanced upon someone whose record showed they had last consulted 15 years ago, at which time they were already 98 years old. But in a purely demand-led system, such discovery would only be by chance. I believe we never knowingly failed to send the records of someone who had left us back to the FPC for deregistration, but that assumes we knew.

Once you had an age-sex register, you could quickly spot such people, at least by age, and check that they were still alive. So, perversely, once you had constructed the register, at your own expense, you were then under a moral and professional obligation to find and report such aged ghosts to a presumably grateful FPC. Improving your practice cost you money, and then lost you more.

Like many other practices, we used our age-sex register as the master registration index, and for our preventive medicine programme, but it was hard work and prone to inaccuracy. Nationally, computers eventually superseded them across the whole of general practice.

Manual disease registers were different again, based on specific conditions rather than age and sex. In 1979, we designed a register based on the ingenious Copeland–Chatterson edge-punch cards. "Cope–Chat" cards came with a row of holes punched around all four sides, and then overprinted with a text of your design to indicate the purpose assigned to each hole.

For example, one hole in ours meant the patient was male,[132] another that they had diabetes, a third represented raised blood pressure, a fourth epilepsy, and so on.

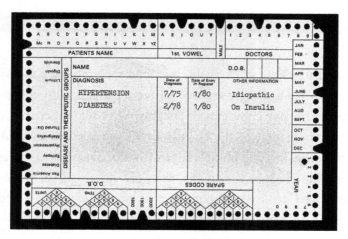

Example of one of our Cope–Chat edge-punch cards.

---

[132] Space was at a premium and we saved a precious hole here; if they were not marked as male we could assume they were female!

A hand punch was used to clip away the edge of a hole to indicate its characteristic was positive; so, for a patient with diabetes, we would clip the diabetes hole. If we took a stack of the cards and slipped a knitting needle through the hole for males, and another through the hole for diabetes, the cards for males with diabetes fell out of the pack.

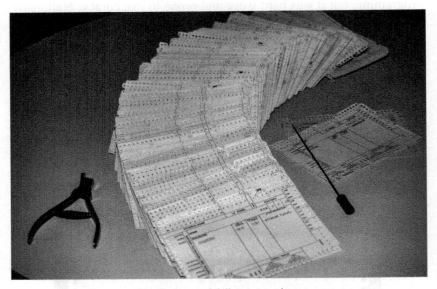

Our disease and follow-up register.

If we used that little stack again, this time spearing the epilepsy hole, in moments we had the names of all male patients with epilepsy and diabetes within our thousands of patients. We could, of course, do this for any combination of the characteristics we had assigned. A great advantage was that the numbers were small compared to the age-sex register. The chronic conditions we were interested in consistently only involved 10–15% of our practice population. The Cope–Chat edge-punch cards were perfect for our purpose.

As a rule, patients with chronic diseases such as those we put on the disease register required regular follow-up. One difficulty was helping them remember when to attend. We hit on the simple idea that it should take place in the month of their birthday, an easy aide-memoire for the patient and a means of effortlessly spreading our workload through the year. Nonetheless, we wanted a follow-up register to ensure clinical reviews were happening as planned. We realised we could incorporate this on the back of our edge-punch cards, so the follow-up and disease registers worked in conjunction.

We could easily see, for example, which of our male patients with diabetes had not attended for review in September as expected, and we could do that with just a stack of cards and two knitting needles. In the example card shown here, the patient was scheduled for review in June and December. In 1981 they had seen the nurse on 2 June. In 1982, there was a phone consultation on 5 January (perhaps a recall), after which they saw me on 3 February, 3 July and 11 December.

Follow-up chart on the back of a patient's disease register card.

I doubt ours was the first use of such cards by GPs, but as far as I know it was the only one that incorporated an integrated disease register, follow-up system, and recall register all on one card.

Our edge-punch cards gave us an organisational ability which we had never possessed before, transforming our management of continuing illness. Together with the age-sex register for preventive care, we felt for the first time that we had a grip on the three broad aspects of our clinical work. However, no sooner had we arrived at this point than the first computers became available for early adopters, and we turned from our manual systems to developing electronic ones.

INFORMATION SYSTEMS: THE EARLY DIGITAL YEARS

DEVELOPING COMPUTER SYSTEMS

In 1969, Intel, the US corporation announced the development of its 4004 chip, the world's first universal, single-chip microprocessor. It packed 2300 transistors into an area of silicon 3 mm × 4 mm. It had the equivalent computing power of the first general-purpose programmable computer, ENIAC,[133] which in 1946 contained 17 600 vacuum tubes and weighed 30 tonnes.[134]

When microcomputers became commercially available from the end of the 1970s,[135] some GPs bought machines and developed their own programs. A notable example was David Ferguson in Scotland, who wrote a system in BASIC[136] for his Commodore PET 4032. In 1983, his software was adopted by the Scottish Home and Health Department as the basis for the General Practice Administration System for Scotland and made available free to all Scottish practices.

Other noteworthy projects by GPs were those of Alan Dean, whose design became the VAMP system; Tim Benson, who created the Abies system; and David Staples and Peter Sowerby, who together

---

[133] Electronic Numerical Integrator And Computer, one of the earliest electronic general-purpose computers.

[134] Britain's top-secret Colossus computer was earlier, beginning work on cracking Germany's Lorenz cyphers at Bletchley Park in February 1944, but Colossus was not a multipurpose machine.

[135] The first three microcomputers were launched in 1997: the Commodore PET; Apple II; and TRS-80. All three had forms of BASIC as their primary programming language.

[136] Beginners' All-purpose Symbolic Instruction Code, a simple high-level computer programming language that uses familiar English words. It was designed for beginners and was formerly used widely.

developed EMIS. These were all successful commercial concerns that expanded to be the leading general practice systems of their day.

By 2001, 97% of English GPs had a computer on their consulting room desk, compared to less than 10% of hospital specialists.[137]

I was another early adopter of GP microcomputing. I first caught the bug in 1980, dabbling with one of Clive Sinclair's tiny ZX80 "home computers", so named not because of the date of its production but rather its Z80 chip. Much was the excitement when owners connected this small wedge of white and blue plastic to their television!

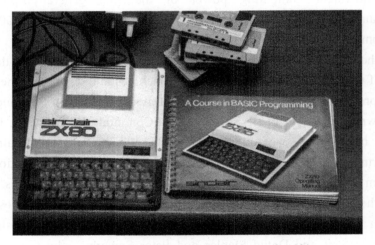

The Sinclair ZX80, my first computer in 1980.

I still bear the emotional scars of frustration from failing at "Moon Lander"; I usually approached too fast, only to crash and burn. Chastened, I was then too hesitant and ran out of fuel; the result was the same. I still have the ZX80, complete with original manuals, case slightly damaged, ever hopeful that the market will pick up. I should have kept the box.

---

[137] Benson T (2001). Why British GPs use computers and hospital doctors do not. *Proc AMIA Symp*, 42–46. [online] Available from: http://tinyurl.com/jfm7yof (accessed 9 January 2017).

But it showed me the relevant potential of computers. You could make them do things, useful things you could do no other way, and I had things at work I wanted to do. I was discussing all this with our practice nurse, Jean, when she suggested I got one of those new Commodore PET things. I had never heard of them. I remember the flashbulb moment; I remember where we were standing, even the directions we were facing. Neither of us could know how pivotal her comment would be for me. Within a few weeks, I had bought a Commodore PET 4032; a proper office machine with its little green screen, keyboard, separate drive for two 720-kilobyte floppy disks, and a dot matrix printer. That all cost £2200,[138] a sum I could set off against tax as a business expense, but there was no financial help from the NHS.

There were almost no off-the-shelf programs available at that time for computers. Anyone who bought a computer expected to have to learn how to program it using BASIC, a language originally created in 1964 as an easy introduction to programming for non-mathematicians. I enrolled for computer evening classes at Northampton College, where we all nervously typed our tentative lines of code into terminals attached to the college's mainframe computer sitting in an air-conditioned room elsewhere. The class was all right as an introduction, but developing your skills required buying a suitable computer, sitting down in front of it, and getting on with writing programs. For those so inclined, usually men, it was an exhilarating and addictive experience that fathered a generation of computer widows.

I wrote some simple initial applications, but what I wanted was a computer by my desk, with the patients' records accessible during consulting sessions. The available commercial systems were only for back-office administrative support and in any case, as in most other practices at that time, my partners quite sensibly did not want to jump

---

[138] This was equivalent to £7100 in 2014 when inflated by the RPI.

into the toy box with me and develop computer systems. So, in 1981, I drew up a detailed design brief and Dave Watts, a friend of Allan Leroy, sat in my house for countless evenings producing an incredible program for me at very modest cost.

At that time, we were also in the throes of developing the practice building, and the architect Peter Aldington agreed to design the furniture for my consulting room. He knew my interest in woodwork, so his only condition was that if he designed it, I had to make it! From him it was predictably clever and complex. A cylinder of over 40 layers of stacked Baltic birch plywood, with each layer made up of four pieces of differing design; it took me six months to complete. The computer sat on top, there was a drawer for the printer and paper, and a bottom compartment for the disk drives. His idea was that by making such an obvious item of the cabinet, it would draw attention away from the threatening computer, which was a very new addition to doctors' consulting rooms anywhere. In fact, I was probably one of the first GPs in the country to have one beside my desk. And his idea worked. Years later, many patients remembered the cabinet while having forgotten that I had a computer.

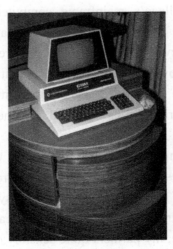

The Commodore PET 4032 and cabinet.

I was thrilled with the computer system. It held a summary record for each of the 2500 patients registered with me. I could search and sort the information in any way I wanted, almost instantly. I could also print repeat prescriptions because it held the necessary details for all my patients on repeat medication. I could list patients with certain diseases at the press of a few buttons and see who had not come for review last month. So-called office computers could not yet run two programs simultaneously, so Dave's software included a bridge that allowed me to enter into his system strings of any additional data I liked about each consultation. Then, when I closed his program, the lines of data were saved automatically to disk, and later could be read by other programs, such as the workload analysis application I wrote myself.

There was insufficient space for narrative records about each consultation, but at the time I did not want that facility in any case.[139] But for the first time, the essential record of any of my patients was instantly available at my desk. There were very few GPs indeed in the country with such functionality, and Dave and I were very proud of the system.

Despite meeting all the elements of my lengthy brief, the whole system only took up two 720-kilobyte floppy discs, one for the programs and the other for the database. By way of comparison, the smallest amount of memory available on my iPhone today is 16 gigabytes, or 16 million kilobytes. Today's programmers are spoilt for storage capacity, and I wonder if many could repeat Dave's feat.

The biggest "extra" was the postdating of repeat prescriptions. During my training, Chris Elliott-Binns taught me to use carbon paper to issue several postdated prescriptions when I saw a patient, enough to last until they needed seeing again. Now I could do it automatically with just a few keystrokes, using the FP10 (Comp) continuous

---

[139] It would be another decade before even the best commercial GP systems moved from summaries to full consultation text.

prescription paper just released by the DoH. In fact, we had obtained a few sheets before the release date for coding purposes so we were ready when it became fully available.

At the end of an appointment, the patient and I would agree when we would meet for the next routine review. A single key press selected the duration of each prescription in months, (that was usually two months, but could be any number I liked); another selected the number of prescriptions, (usually three if I was making each prescription of two-month duration, giving a total of six months' treatment); and pressing a third key printed them, each one dated three days before the previous one was due to run out, to allow for chemists shutting at weekends. All the patient had to do was to store them carefully and take them in sequence to the chemist. In any case, some chemists kept the scripts for them. When the last one was running out, patients knew it was time to come again for review, another beneficial feature. If they wanted to come before then, of course they were free to do so, but that was now their choice, not mine.

Patients liked it for its simplicity and convenience. Receptionists, none of whom had clinical or pharmacological training, appreciated not having to take messages for repeat prescriptions, a potentially dangerous practice in any case. I liked it because I had few if any repeat prescriptions to sign outside consulting sessions, and as a bonus, my recall system operated automatically. Everyone won.

I used my consulting room system very happily for three years, neither the design nor the programming requiring alteration throughout that time. But things moved on, commercial systems improved, and we all realised the time had come to install one throughout the practice. We chose the then market leader, the VAMP system, on condition that the company added my postdated repeat prescription system.

It was installed in January 1986, complete with eight terminals, seven printers and a tape streamer for backups, and with postdated repeat prescriptions now an integral part of the VAMP software nationally.

By October, we were using it for all our administrative indexes. Gleefully, we put our manual registers in the loft for a few months – just in case – before shredding them.

For the first time, we could enter data in any of the clinical rooms during consultations, dramatically reducing duplication. We still used a Lloyd-Hamel appointment system as VAMP still had nothing comparable to offer, nor could it handle free text records of individual consultations. We therefore still needed to operate dual systems, the computer and manual records, which was very inefficient, time-consuming, and prone to inaccuracy. For our staff, it was the busiest time in the history of the practice. We comforted ourselves with the analogy that we had to climb the mountain before we could slide down the other side into a peaceful valley. But it was a considerable mountain.

PAPER-FREE CONSULTING AT LAST

When, in 1992, we moved to our new building in King Edward Road we wanted to make the big change, to work without paper records. VAMP did not have that capability, while the emerging EMIS system had electronic appointments and could also hold consultation textual records. And so we made the change and completed the transfer from paper records to electronic ones.

Of course, in reality there was still paper. Our goal was to "consult without recourse to paper records", and in that we were successful. I doubt any practice was truly paper-free. For one thing, hospitals almost everywhere continued to write to GPs on A4 paper, an odd thing to do considering GP record envelopes were approximately A5 in size. There were honourable exceptions. A few hospitals used sensibly sized paper, some even with space on one side for the GP referral and the specialist's reply on the other. That some could do it

merely exposed the disdain of most hospitals for the needs of GPs. I
know a GP who was so upset by this lack of consideration that he
wrote a few referral letters to hospitals on A3 paper, to make the
point.

Each sheet of A4 paper required folding twice to fit the Edwardian
envelope. And as time passed, so the quantities of correspondence and
investigation results increased, with more and more paper stuffed into
overstretched envelopes. Among a significant minority of practices,
we stopped using the paper records, so we were even less inclined to
thin them by removing paper no longer required. They became a
repository for hospital correspondence and investigation results, most
of which were obsolete and of no value whatsoever.

The solution was to scan incoming hospital correspondence,
include the scanned image in the patient's electronic record, and then
shred the paper version.[140] Scanning was a real breakthrough not only
in storage terms but also because it meant we had convenient access to
hospital reports within the electronic records used during
consultations. Gone were phone calls to receptionists, asking them to
bring the patient's paper record so we could wade through that store of
fossilised hospital correspondence. They had to waste time finding the
record and more time bringing them to our rooms while we twiddled
our thumbs and chatted aimlessly with the patient, who might well be
anxious and rightly puzzled the doctor did not have the information to
hand. Scanning the letters straight into the medical record removed all
that nonsense and EMIS as a company was very helpful in facilitating
the process.

Yes, computers can assist acute care, but they are essential for
practical programmes of preventive medicine and the management of
chronic conditions. In the 1970s, it was just about possible to manage
these services with card registers. In practice, it was prohibitively

---

[140] Our computer was backed up every night, and in any case, the paper
originals were kept by the hospital.

time-consuming. Computers allow you to identify cohorts of patients quickly, write to them, and invite them for recall or a screening procedure, or for any other reason. And then you can use the system to monitor the care provided by the practice, and adjust operational plans as needed to achieve better results.

By 2006, we were using the WWW to access national and international databases for education and diagnostic information; we had our own Intranet and were using electronic communications both inside and outside the practice. Our patients were arranging appointments and repeat prescriptions online, just as they were accessing our website for various services and information. We could be sure of only one thing. The pace of change was accelerating, and within a few years, these achievements would seem very modest indeed.

MORE PLAYFUL INNOVATION

With our major computer installation in place, we could return to playful innovation, though now with a much larger box of bricks. Like many other practices, we tweaked our system to suit our purposes better.

But we hit a snag. One of the essential requirements for Fellowship by Assessment of the RCGP was to have patient records with you on a home visit. We could take a printout from the computer, but that would not work for an emergency when we were already away from the practice. We needed a readily available electronic record at a time before we could access them at the practice remotely via the WWW. Thanks to Mark, a son now conveniently studying computing at university, we developed Pocket EMIS, a system for downloading an encrypted summary record for all our patients onto a Psion palmtop computer. Despite holding over 8000 patient summaries, it was far more secure than paper records. If you dropped it in the street or left it at the patient's house, the encrypted files were inaccessible to anyone without the password, which was also encrypted. With this in the pocket of the duty doctor, the most essential information about any patient was always available, no matter where the doctor took the call.

It was ingenious, and people at national conferences were incredulous. In reality, it was far less useful than we had imagined. We quickly realised just how little historical information you need to take on a visit. It is usually easier just to ask the patient, and advocates of the national electronic record may yet come to the same conclusion. There are exceptions of course, but the vast majority of patients seeking acute care can answer questions. The great majority of them are not drunk, psychotic, or unconscious. People known to be at a particular risk need to take particular precautions. As an example, my granddaughter in Zimbabwe has an anaphylactic reaction to bee stings, so she wears a MedicAlert bracelet at all times, which is recognised all over the world, supported by an international database, and engraved with her specific problem. For her, that is a superior solution to any national electronic record system, particularly as it is a cool fashion accessory that she is permitted to wear at school.

Health education presented a clear use for computers. It could ask the person a branching questionnaire, collect and analyse the answers, and produce a report that advised what they could do to improve their health. BUPA has used such systems for decades, and we went to see their system in operation. James, one of my brothers and also a GP, had produced a program in the 1980s for his own practice. It was a great success with his patients, and we installed a copy as well; over 600 of our patients used it. Over 10 years later, we developed a new system, making use of what were inevitably more advanced technologies, such as touchscreens, more powerful computers, and a broader range of evidence-based information. And, handily, Mark now needed a project for his computer science dissertation. His system was also very popular and received a 97% approval rating from its users.

Another of his projects was a management information system we called Magpie.[141] All the necessary data were exported overnight from our EMIS system to a more flexible Microsoft Access database. There, we could use the data in whatever way we wanted, and quite independently from EMIS, which was a much more rigid, limited system when it came to non-clinical tasks. Magpie was a remarkable program and a great success. It gave us flexible tools to analyse and manage our work at least a year before similar systems were made available nationally to facilitate the QOF.

With our EMIS clinical system, Magpie for practice management and clinical audit, Internet access, our website and Intranet, and even Pocket EMIS, we had all the information we needed, where and when we wanted it.

Except, what if EMIS was not available? We were consulting using just electronic records, so if EMIS shut down for any reason, we would have a very real problem: no appointment system to know who to expect, and no records with which to consult anyway. To counter this, Mark included in Magpie's facilities a summary of every patient's record, an expanded version of that used in Pocket EMIS. These were regularly updated overnight, stored on our second independent server, and available throughout the practice via our Intranet. As an emergency system, this was fantastic. We could be up and running with our alternative record system only 10 or 15 minutes after EMIS crashed.

Even the EMIS company was surprised we could do it, just as they had been with Pocket EMIS. (A name, incidentally, they said we could not use if we distributed it, because of copyright, or some restriction like that. Later they produced their own version.) In reality, the greatest benefit was the reassurance to staff and clinicians of

---

[141] Obviously, magpies are known for hoarding things, and in our case that was data. Less obviously, it was also named in honour of our manager Maggie, though I am not absolutely sure she appreciated the association with a bird, no matter how clever and adaptable magpies are.

knowing that we had such a facility of resilience. EMIS was a very reliable system, and we only used our emergency record system on a few occasions. But when we needed it, it was terrific, a wonderful get-out-of-jail card.

It is because of the computer that general practice can now fulfil its potential as the base unit of managed population care within the NHS. It was simply not possible beforehand. Many further developments have occurred since those early days in the 1980s and 1990s, and in some ways, practices have been overwhelmed by the additional tasks and expectations computing has brought. And there are more pressures to come, as an ever-greater amount of medical care rightly moves back from hospitals into the community. The future of the NHS depends on practices being able to deal with those challenges.

AT THE CUTTING EDGE

I think there is a world market for maybe five computers.

Thomas Watson, chairman of IBM, 1943

General practice changed with the coming of computers in the 1980s. It is difficult now to realise their effect, opening an extraordinary range of opportunities. While the previous two chapters described the evolution of GP systems, and ours in particular, this one describes some of the national research and development projects we were involved with between 1989 and 2005. For a few years, we were at the cutting edge, a leading practice in the construction of some of the NHS information infrastructure we now take for granted.

Between 1989 and 1992, we were the practice at the heart of the NHS Open Systems Interconnection (OSI) demonstrator.[142] The project took place in our health district; after three years, the health authority invited the head of the NHS to come and see the results. The idea was to get computers from different manufacturers, using different operating systems, to communicate using open systems technology. It was all very new indeed. Leading experts from far and wide said it was impossible, yet here was a demonstration of it happening for the first time.

***

Tension is in the air! How often do demonstrations of new technology go wrong, or simply not work at all? For that matter, how often do they go right?

---

[142] OSI is a standard for worldwide communication that defines a networking framework using protocols in seven layers. Once expected to become the universal communication standard, it has been superseded and now serves as a teaching model for all other protocols.

Around my desk crowd the most senior officers from the health authority – the chairman, the chief executive, and his number two, Mike Sobanja. From the project team are the manager, Keith Oswin, the programmer who does the smart stuff, David Morgan, and me – the so-called user representative. Duncan Nichol, Chief Executive Officer (CEO) of the NHS and guest of honour, is sitting in the patient's chair by my desk. He seems genuinely interested in watching the first of these pioneering communications within his NHS.

First, it is the pathology lab's turn. Its minicomputer, which uses one operating system, sends a fictitious test report about Duncan Nichol to the microcomputer on my desk running VAMP and a different operating system. Success. Then there is a message for him from the A & E department, which uses a unique system peculiar to just a few units in the country. We encourage the CEO to use my computer to book himself an outpatient appointment. The hospital's mainframe replies instantly with an automated, confirmatory response. Finally, he receives a message from one of David's techy friends in France, who is using a different system again. He congratulates Duncan Nichol on a successful OSI demonstrator project.

That last item seems particularly dramatic for the mundane reason that, of course, it is in French. But it is genius on the part of David; it startles to make the point. The head of the NHS is witnessing the very start of the open systems that now we take for granted. Different computer hardware, using different operating systems are talking to each other in different languages from different countries. Before today they could not. It is as if separate parts of the NHS have been speaking their own languages, but now there is an invisible, automatic translator.

***

That game-changing watershed was so important that it needs putting in context. By the end of the 1980s, the strategic development

231 · PRACTICE MATTERS

of GP computer systems was a mess. Although far in advance of anything available to most hospital clinicians, they were also twisting practices into an ever-tightening administrative knot. The systems were good enough to allow practices to expand their services into preventive medicine and chronic disease management. They were good enough for many back-office, administrative tasks and to be of real value in the consultation as a partial medical record. But they were not sufficiently comprehensive to stand alone without the traditional paper records.

Neither paper nor computers could do everything on their own. As we saw in the last chapter, we needed both. One consequence was that they each had to duplicate a lot of material, to be entered manually. Already busy practices were getting busier, largely because of the inefficiency of these duplicate systems and a shortage of staff. The level of financial reimbursement for staff remained that established in the 1960s, well before computers had been invented, and did not cater for the increased workload resulting from preventive medicine and chronic disease management. Policymakers failed to understand. They felt computers should reduce work (true, for individual tasks), so there would be no need for additional staff (false, if they dramatically increase the number of tasks to be undertaken).

The real point was that computers allowed a massive expansion of the work, awakening the slumbering giant, the service's exciting, latent potential for population-based healthcare. But for that to thrive, three things were required: (1) enhanced software; (2) more resources; and (3) the ability for different computer systems to efficiently exchange information. The OSI demonstrator project addressed the third of those.

At that time, many were surprised that computers from different manufacturers could not communicate. The best-known example was the incompatibility between Apple and the many clones of the IBM personal computer, but it applied equally elsewhere, including microcomputers, minicomputers, and mainframes used within health authorities and hospitals. This lack of connectivity meant that hospitals, practices, health authorities, and FHSAs had to communicate by printing information out of one computer and retyping it into another.

Looking back, it beggars belief. But to offer a milestone on the path of systems development, on 6 August 1991, nearer the end than the beginning of the cutting-edge OSI demonstrator project I have just described, the WWW was made available to the public for the first time. For almost half of my career, the WWW did not exist.

Within the NHS, the glimpse of the obvious was that for computer systems to replace paper ones they would have to communicate directly by electronic means. One solution would be for the DoH to choose a single manufacturer for all machines used within the service. But that directly contradicted government policy for England and Wales,[143] which was to use market forces between suppliers to encourage the evolution of systems. The market horses had already bolted, and a multiplicity of different systems existed. They just could not talk to one another.

Given the enormity of the NHS, and the ever-changing hardware and operating systems used in different places, the only practical possibility was to use internationally agreed communication standards. This was hardly a new idea. For example, international telephone calls were possible because relevant companies in different countries using different equipment worked to recognised communication standards.

By 1989, the NHS had decided to pilot electronic communications within a health district.[144] The project was set up in Northampton and funded by the Department of Trade and Industry (DTI) (now the

---

[143] As I have already said, Scotland chose the opposite approach, supplying a single system to all its practices.
[144] NHS OSI Demonstrator Project (1990–1992). A three-year project for the development of OSI-based computer networks to enhance patient care in the NHS.

Department for Innovation, Universities and Skills), the Oxford Region and Northampton Health Authority. Our practice was invited to be the practice involved with our VAMP system, communicating with two hospital wards, the admissions department, pathology laboratory, the department of surgery, and the A & E department. These different sites all used incompatible hardware and operating systems. The project was developing the necessary technology to allow them to communicate.

Our task within the project team was to represent the users of the relevant computer systems; everyone else was very much on the technical side. Such an imbalance could have swamped the project, leaving the techies thrilled but the users with ingenious sets of wire and silicon and little in the way of practical functionality.

One example will suffice to make the point. Of particular interest to the practice was the electronic transfer of pathology results. The existing position was not only farcical but potentially dangerous. The laboratory's computer systems would analyse the test results and then print them out on paper in the laboratory office. Every day batches of these were then sent by NHS courier (for reasons of confidentiality) to the relevant practices throughout the health district, which covered half of Northamptonshire.

In our case, they would then be sorted by receptionists into the correct piles for the doctors who requested the tests, and distributed to the relevant doctors' desks. If we wanted the results placed in the computer record, then we scribbled on them and that would be typed into the computer, usually by a lay receptionist with no clinical training. If we wanted the staff to contact the patient, we would scribble another message on the form. After we had checked them, they would be collected up again by receptionists, any messages phoned through to patients, any results we had specified typed into the patient's computer record, and then the paper filed in the record envelopes.

Within the project, the hospital and technical people saw the solution as quite straightforward. They would transfer the result electronically straight from the laboratory's computer to another stand-alone machine in the practice, which would automatically print them out. Apparently, this would be a successful outcome.

In a way it would be, demonstrating data transfer between different systems. It would even be of some trivial help to the laboratory (no printing) and health authority (no courier). And for us, it would provide the results more quickly, but do nothing else other than to replace the courier's visit with the intermittent screech of a hidden dot matrix printer within the supposedly serene calm of our open-plan office and reception area.

What we needed was something far more useful and far more ambitious. We were not so much interested in the technology as to make use of the opportunities it presented. We wanted the pathology results to go straight from the pathology laboratory's computer directly to the doctor's terminal for checking, and then directly into the patient's computer records. That would not be easy.

In the first place, there were technical issues. It required using numbers rather than the text of a printed result. So, we wanted 9 to be recognisable to our computer as a number, of being one more than 8, rather than a word – nine, which is just a string of four characters. By integrating the numeric result, VAMP could then compare the 9 to, say, a previous 14, and know that the new one was lower. With text, it could not do that.

Once we had checked the results on a terminal anywhere in the building, we needed to be able to take appropriate action on screen. Perhaps a message for the patient to be read out by the receptionist from her screen when they phoned; perhaps forwarding the result and a message to a colleague within VAMP. And eventually, as and when we instructed it, the system would automatically file the results in the patient's computer record.

This insistence by the practice for a much more challenging outcome caused a significant intake of breath when I put it to the project's board. It would require substantial, unexpected work, not least from VAMP, our benevolent but nonetheless commercial GP system supplier. To the immense credit of the project and VAMP, we got all we asked for, becoming the first practice in the UK, and probably in Europe, to have the groundbreaking facility of integrating investigation results from incompatible external systems using internationally recognised data transfer protocols.

But, as I have said, the OSI project did not stop with pathology results. We also received a report following any of our patient's attendance at A & E. Again, that department used its own software and operating system. If the hospital admitted one of our patients who broke their hip on an icy path, we already knew about it when their relation phoned the next morning. Similarly, when patients left the surgical wards, we had received their automated discharge summary before they got home.

Overall, the project was a success. It was the beginning of the NHS network, of the electronic communications, and the system interoperability that is now just assumed. It was a pioneering, technical project, but it kept in the foreground, just, the people who use the systems.

***

If the OSI demonstrator was primarily technical, with few direct benefits for patients, then another project we were involved in was considerably different. In 2001, we were invited to take part in another national pilot, the Electronic Transfer of Prescriptions (ETP) project, which explored moving prescriptions around the NHS electronically rather than on paper. It used the NHS network we were involved with during the OSI demonstrator 10 years earlier. The ETP appeared to offer tremendous benefits to patients on long-term medication, but I suspect the NHS hierarchy was more concerned with the logistical issues of transporting half a billion paper prescriptions round the NHS each year. Perhaps I am unduly cynical.

Nationally, each paper prescription had to pass from the practice, where it was often still copied out by non-clinical staff from a computer record, to the patient, who would take it to the pharmacist for dispensing. After that, the prescription went to the Prescription Pricing Authority (PPA) in Newcastle-upon-Tyne (now called NHS Prescription Services) where its details would once more be rekeyed into the PPA computer system for processing.[145] That assumed, of course, that the typist there, like the pharmacist beforehand, could read the doctor's handwriting. To my knowledge, there is no record of how many clinical and clerical errors occurred with this extraordinarily cumbersome and labour-intensive system, but it would be naïve to argue that there were none.

From the perspective of the patients on repeat medication, the system was equally ridiculous. They had to contact their practice to order fresh supplies and then wait to collect the prescription and go to the chemist to hand it in. Another delay, perhaps even requiring them to return later to collect their medication. And there was pressure on practices from the DoH to continue issuing prescriptions monthly, perhaps for the rest of the patients' lives, even though in our case we could demonstrate lower than average prescribing costs using prescriptions of two or three months' duration. On top of all that, patients had to remember when to attend at their practice for review.

By now there was email and the WWW; there had to be a better way.

Our involvement was within one of three NHS pilot projects that tested different approaches. Happily, the one to which we were

---

[145] The main functions of the PPA were to calculate and make payments for amounts due to pharmacists and appliance contractors, and calculate amounts due to GPs, for supplying drugs and appliances prescribed under the NHS. The PPA was abolished in 2006.

attached seemed to offer a Rolls-Royce service to patients while fully meeting the desired technical goal. It was the only pilot to do that. Its peculiarity was that it only involved a single GP computer system supplier, EMIS, and a single pharmacy, which operated from a distribution centre in Leeds. Perhaps those tight constraints contributed to it being the most successful of the three pilots.

Later I saw a much larger, but otherwise similar, arrangement working at the Southern California division of Kaiser Permanente. There a 24-hour automated pharmacy used robots to dispense and post to patients' homes 66% of the prescriptions for the Kaiser Permanente population of 3.2 million people living in that lower half of the state, and all from a single pharmacy.

Within our project, patients could organise their prescriptions by phone, email, or online. Items went by special postal delivery to any address the patient liked in the UK, usually their home but if necessary a neighbour or their place of work. There was no charge for this service because the saving in having no high-street outlets offset the pharmacy's additional costs.

Because the project automatically synchronised the pharmacy's records with those of the GP, the pharmacist was aware of the patient's up-to-date repeat medication as well as their review date at the practice. Consequently, the pharmacy could remind patients when it was time for their review and any changes in medication by the GP were immediately and automatically transmitted to update the pharmacy records.

For many patients, it was an attractive option. A study within the project found that 99% of patients using the system found home delivery to be helpful, and 94% of those choosing to ask the pharmacy to prompt them for repeats appreciated that facility. Of particular interest to the practice was that 95% of our patients who used the service ordered directly from the pharmacy, and received prescriptions to their door, without having to contact the practice themselves, or having to go to a chemist at all.

The electronic requests from the pharmacy to authorise prescriptions came to the GP within our EMIS system. There was a facility for the pharmacy to query items or ask questions, and for the GP to respond, all done electronically. When prescriptions were agreed, it was simply a matter of the GP entering a four-digit security code for their electronic signature (just once for each batch). The prescriptions went to the pharmacy across the NHS network; the first use of encrypted clinical data and digital signatures passing across the network, and another first in Europe.

Did it make a difference? It was rated either "excellent" or "good" by 99% of those using it. Has there ever been a more enthusiastic response from patients to an NHS pilot project? Over 600 of our patients used it and felt it simpler and more convenient. The most frequent complaint was that the post delivered the items too early in the morning.

But a more significant disadvantage for some patients – those that chose not to use it – was that many people like being able to go to their local pharmacy. By its very nature, this particular project did not allow that, although patients could use a Freephone number to call the pharmacy and speak to a pharmacist at any time. It is probably also true that those who tried it did not find the lack of a local pharmacy a problem. They could still go to one if they wanted to, even when using this system, though I think very few did for their repeat medication. (The project did not encompass one-off prescriptions for short-term, acute problems.) Nonetheless, that the pharmacy was remote was an issue for some potential users.

For the practices, the clerical task of processing repeat prescriptions for the patients involved ceased to exist for 95% of repeat medication requests. Our staff loved it. We issued over 15 000 electronic prescriptions during the project, and many other practices became involved in different areas of the country, meaning many thousands of patients were gaining benefit. It was a safer system. It could only issue prescription items that a doctor had put into the patient's record. The chance of an unnoticed transcription error by an untrained receptionist was eliminated, as was the misinterpretation of a doctor's scribble on a handwritten prescription.

For the NHS, the project resolved the problem of transporting paper prescriptions around the system. It happened automatically and without the use of paper or rekeying at all. The pharmacy and the PPA could process the prescriptions electronically from beginning to end. In this project, paper prescriptions, handwritten or printed, were a thing of the past.

In short, everyone benefited. It was by far the most successful NHS computer project we were ever involved with, producing real benefits for everyone and providing valuable technical and practical information. Unfortunately, at the end of the project, the ETP pilots were stopped in their tracks by the notoriously unsuccessful and costly Connecting for Health IT programme for the NHS. The health service then took 12 years to develop and roll out the resulting full-blown, national system for ETP.

That uncaring decision made me furious. It swept aside technical excellence and the substantial benefits enjoyed by several thousand particularly needy patients taking part across the UK, and all for the sake of central convenience and control – an act of policymakers' arrogant self-centredness. Not much there about putting the patient first. Clearly, it was correct to use the pilot projects to help develop a national system, but it was wrong to remove a fully functioning service of excellence before its replacement was available 12 years later.

THE EVOLVING TEAM

Coming together is a beginning, staying together is progress, and working together is a success.

Henry Ford

The number of NHS GPs has risen over recent decades, but there has been an explosion in practice staff. An example will not only illustrate the point but also indicate why this change occurred.

In 1973, our practice could be summarised as follows: three doctors plus a trainee (the training scheme started in 1971); three part-time, untrained receptionists; and three attached community nurses who called in occasionally (district nurse, health visitor, and midwife).

Our task was to provide acute care, child preventive work, and midwifery to 9500 patients, 24 hours a day, every day of the year. We managed 96% of consultations without referral to hospital.

The practice worked from a poorly adapted, four-storey Edwardian house, and used no information systems at all other than unstructured paper records and an appointment book.

It was a different age: before the WWW, email, mobile phones, and social media; a time of writing letters in ink, posting them, and waiting; of many patients having neither car nor phone. The word "team" was for sport and recreation but not general practice. Some tinkered with it, talking about a primary care team as if primary care was general practice, but with a few notable exceptions (the William Budd Health Centre in 1952 being one) never with any organisational justification.

For us, there was certainly the partnership, an entity of practical and legal significance, but it was not a team in the sense accepted now within organisational management. The two or three receptionists were part-time employees necessary to command the waiting room and, together with our wives, to take messages; and there were the newly attached community nurses, their work invaluable to patients but operating within a parallel universe. They only occasionally made intergalactic sorties to our mother earth for brief negotiations, while sadly we never even thought of going to them.

And that was our world, the world of a pretty typical general practice.

In 1975, we made a decisive breakthrough by employing a secretary. Until then, most referral letters were written by hand. Any typing was undertaken at home, at first by one of the receptionists and later by the wife of a GP trainee. That is why we had a small, blue, portable typewriter; so that anyone who could type and was willing to do so could take it home to type letters in the evening. But even this much demonstrated the advantage of having a proper typist. When she and her husband moved on, we employed our first part-time secretary. Jane made a great impact, her value and personality planting a seed, a glimpse of the obvious; everyone could benefit if we got other people to do some things for us. To that point, a very real weakness in most general practices was a culture of the doctors doing almost everything themselves.

In 1977, that seed germinated and we employed Jean, our very own nurse. It was a distinctly odd thing for a practice to do. We created our first treatment room out of the small Edwardian bathroom on the first floor and with Jean installed there the practice never looked back. Doctors, secretary, practice nurse, receptionists, and attached community midwife, health visitor, and district nurse. At least we now had the people for a team, but it would be some years before we behaved like one.

**

By the time we left Billing Road just 17 years later, we had expanded considerably. We had a full-time practice manager supported by a deputy, filing clerk, medical secretary, information officer, computer manager, and seven receptionists with their administrator. We had 4 practice nurses who between them worked 76 hours per week, with one of them employed specifically to visit older patients in their homes to offer a health check. Our employed staff moved from about 1.5 whole time equivalents in 1974 to 12.5 two decades later.

And it did not stop there. By 2004, the entire team at the practice, including the doctors and community staff, numbered 42. Two healthcare assistants supported 4 practice-employed nurses; a total of 14 administration and support staff included receptionists, and computer and audit staff. Two full-time health visitors with their clerical assistant, a district nursing team of three, a midwife, and two psychiatric nurses together made up the community staff, all of whom worked full-time, with their base in offices within our practice (except for the psychiatric nurses).

There was a mental health graduate worker, a counsellor, a GP trainee (now politically rebadged as a registrar), and our own pharmaceutical adviser to help patients and clinicians alike. And there was the PSG, intentionally distanced from the professional team to preserve its independence, but an important element in our practice community. Despite this impressive team, we were still dealing with the same number of patients as in 1973. Why should this be?

The reasons behind this explosion in personnel, common throughout general practice, reflected several factors. The most important was the extension of general practice to include preventive medicine and chronic disease management within its portfolio. And then, by their presence in the practice, the additional, skilled staff unmasked further opportunities. Practices had developed a virtuous circle. Advanced information systems enabled more and more clinical work to be undertaken, requiring more and more staff, who unmasked further opportunities that in the past had silently glided by unseen.

There were other reasons. An increasingly managed health service created additional administrative work, as did our shift from the ad hoc, reactive service and organised curiosity of the 1970s to the 1990s managed care, audit, reflection, and learning. Finally, such complex, multidisciplinary teams need careful management, and that itself created its own work.

***

What is a team, and in particular, what is a primary healthcare team?

Historically, general practice has struggled in no small part because GPs have not delegated, or acquired the support staff to whom they could do so. When someone asked Thomas Edison why he had a team of 21 assistants, he is reported to have replied: "If I could solve all the problems myself, I would."

By 2004, we had twice as many people in our PHCT as he did, but at least 50% were semiautonomous clinicians, each with their views, priorities, and ways of doing things. Again, about 20% – an overlapping Venn circle – were not employed directly by the practice and so had additional allegiances elsewhere; perhaps stronger ones.

Another difficulty in forming teams in general practice is the enduring difference between clinical and administrative staff. If your role is to support someone else, then it is difficult, though not impossible, to have a peer relationship with them, particularly if they are your boss.

Nonetheless, it is clearly in the best interests of a practice and its patients that those working there should do so as closely and harmoniously as possible, for then their collective endeavour can exceed the individual contributions. PHCTs should not only be teams on paper but teams in practice. A quote usually attributed to Buchholz and Roth says: "Wearing the same shirts doesn't make you a team."

And we did not even wear the same shirts.

Or, as the Scottish-American industrialist Andrew Carnegie put it:

> *Teamwork is the ability to work together toward a common vision. The ability to direct individual accomplishment toward organizational objectives.*

Members of a good team help each other because they believe in the task before them. They may have different skills and personalities, but by working together, their team is more likely to succeed, to build its log raft before the others do, get across the river first and collect the prize. That is a very different picture to the one of general practice described earlier, yet its description throws the essentials of teamwork into sharp relief.

The PHCT is usually taken to mean all those working within or from a general practice to provide healthcare services for the registered population of that practice. Fine, but that does not describe how this disparate group of clinicians and support staff can achieve that objective. It is important to note here the important, practical reason why that definition does not include community pharmacists, dentists, and opticians. The PHCT so defined provides comprehensive, cohesive services for the fundamental, smallest unit of population in the NHS, the practice list of patients. It is not arrogance that excludes the other three disciplines of primary care from that definition; it is that a practice's population is not the inherent focus of their work.

In an average practice such as ours, the PHCT could be quite large, placing another obstacle in the road. Organisational research suggests that effectiveness is often inversely proportional to the size of the team. Small is beautiful, 40 is big.

Fortunately, because of its loose multidisciplinary nature, it is seldom that all members are needed to do the same thing. Small groups form and disburse around a particular task, reminding me of the plumes of hot wax hypnotically rising in a lava lamp. Here the PHCT acts as a resource pool, a matrix of people with specialist knowledge and skills, to be used to form disparate task teams as needed. For task A we need one of these, one of those, and best have one of those others too. It is a concept that makes the best use of the available people, any one of whom may be engaged in several of the task teams at the same time. Sport has few similarities, though perhaps the offensive and defensive teams of American football come close.

MYTEAM

The above appears a very parochial view of the PHCT, one from the practice's perspective. In the future, a more contemporary model might be what we could call the "Myteam", the patient's personal team. In the previous description of the PHCT, there is an empty chair, an absent member. Most descriptions of the PHCT, or of clinical teams anywhere, do not include patients; they try to make organisational sense of a diverse group of professionals delivering a service. But the Myteam construct offers a useful counterpoint.

It has the attraction that we can all picture it very easily. I may have my dentist, my GP, my optician, my osteopath, and of course my chemist and my invaluable helper next door. They have other duties of course, and they belong to other teams, dispersing and transferring as soon as they finish with me. But from my point of view, while they are in Myteam they look after me.

What is interesting is that the members of Myteam change, perhaps frequently. Last month it was my GP and the nurse who took my blood tests, that nice one whose boy goes to the same school as my kids. Today, though, the Myteam has altered a bit, with my consultant now joined by my anaesthetist, and by Beth, my named nurse on the ward. In two weeks, it will shift again, back to my GP and the visiting district nurse, my wife, the team leader, the man from social services I met yesterday but whose name I forget, my daughter, and Jane, the lovely nurse from Marie Curie. Later still? Well, let us worry about that when we get there, but I know Myteam will help me, no matter what.

Myteam is experiential and task-oriented; it forms and reforms as circumstances change, using elements of the available resource pool; in this way, it echoes the PHCT with its matrix management. Because it is more focused and more personal, it is easier to visualise, but the concepts are the same.

Research by Feiger and Schmitt in 1979 found clinical outcomes for patients were better where professionals worked together as teams.[146] Interestingly, they also found results were better the less hierarchical the structure of the team. Perhaps we would have had the flashbulb a bit earlier if Thomas Edison had treated his 21 assistants as peers, and listened more carefully to their ideas, but I may be doing him an injustice.

Hospital work tends to fall naturally into the care of specific conditions and has long offered examples of effective teamwork. Transplant teams, stoma care teams, A & E triage, and the teamwork within ICUs are just examples of this. Furthermore, such teams may stay together for some time, developing their mutual experience and expertise. As a very junior hospital doctor, for nine months I assisted a very distinguished orthopaedic surgeon with most of his NHS and private operations. Much more importantly, he had the same theatre sister throughout, with whom he had worked for some years. He believed speed, and precise technique caused the patient less operative trauma and less chance of infection.

---

[146] Feiger SM, Schmitt MH (1979). Collegiality in interdisciplinary health teams: its measurement and its effects. *Soc Sci Med*, 13A(2): 217–229.

Concentration, anticipation, and precision were essential. After the sister had broken me in, he could once more perform total hip replacements very quickly indeed, without a word said throughout the procedure. Instruments, swabs, and retractors were in the right place at the right time. There was no pause, other than for the acrylic cement to harden. That was teamwork, and it was deeply satisfying.

In the chapter titled "Putting It All into Practice", I describe how our PHCT and patients used small task groups to further the practice's development.

***

The role that has undergone the most change in the last 40 years is that of the receptionists, who have experienced a rollercoaster of change. They saw manual systems sprout and develop, permitting the first dalliances with population care. Those systems and their computerised offspring imposed a tidal surge in work. So, the life of receptionists became harder and harder. They were the administrative backbone of most practices, fighting multiple approaching fronts. The paper records were falling apart at the seams; they had to learn and use additional computer systems; adapt to the increasing use of the telephone by patients; and cope with the expanding clinical work of the practice, including the rise in repeat medication.

All that was in the background. Despite having no clinical training, the priority for receptionists was to arrange the use of the practice's finite appointments as best they could, while being pleasant and helpful to patients. It was a time when overworked, stressed-out receptionists got a bad reputation as being dragons at the door, blocking the way to the beloved doctor. "If only he knew it was me, he would see me at once." I bet that person was a queue jumper anywhere.

I had a profound admiration for our receptionists, multitaskers par excellence. I know I could not have done their job.

Something had to give. Eventually, it was the electronic tide that turned. We had climbed that mountain, and now we were indeed sliding down the other side into greener pastures. At last, we had computers that not only allowed us to do more for our patients but also did more for our staff. They were to have a revolutionary effect on the work of receptionists. The electronic automation of test results was the first snowdrop of their spring. As described earlier, from 1992 our receptionists, uniquely at first, no longer had to deal with pathology results (and there could be over a hundred a day) other than to read the doctor's message to inquiring patients. "All normal." "Please repeat the test in a month." That type of thing, but it was direct from the doctor and not an attempt by the receptionist to interpret a result.

Electronic appointment systems replaced the Lloyd-Hamel appointment book that had served practices all over the country so well. Now receptionists could make appointments from more than one desk at the same time, including rooms at a distance from the reception desk that offered greater confidentiality.[147] Doctors and nurses could book appropriate follow-up appointments before the patient left the consulting room, meaning less work again for the receptionist, who was also helped by the electronic check-in terminals that allowed patients to record their arrival quickly and easily.

The electronic transfer of repeat prescriptions followed, meaning receptionists had fewer of these to deal with. Similarly, their methods of communication with patients and other members of the team changed with internal messaging across our Intranet, and external email via the NHS network. It has been a remarkable four decades for receptionists.

---

[147] A logical progression would come with patients making appointments over the WWW, which is commonplace today.

COMMUNITY NURSES

The members of the PHCT most taxed by the implementation of teamwork were the community staff. Although members of the PHCT, they were usually employed by other organisations and therefore also had to recognise other management lines. Often, they had to work with more than one practice and more than one PHCT, giving them a further sphere of involvement. And to a greater or lesser extent, they may have sensed a reticence to their involvement by the approach of the practice's "home team" of doctors and employed staff.

For example, a busy community nurse might call into the practice and wait patiently for a doctor to be free to speak about their mutual patient, perhaps during a coffee break. Eventually, the doctor appears, probably late for coffee. Perversely, I sometimes hated coffee breaks. Already late, I had only a few minutes, and even those would make me even later for the next patient, who had seen me sheepishly skulking off towards the common room, already after the time of their scheduled appointment. But after two hours I had to have a break, if only for a few minutes.

There was a need to pour coffee, should any remain in the pot; to relax for just a moment. And there was a community nurse who had taken the trouble to come to see me, unnecessarily apologetic for the disturbance, perhaps needing to discuss pressing issues or to ask me to sign an urgent prescription; perhaps to ask me to visit the patient. They understood the pressure, but it would be natural for the nurses to question the whole process. They would be right; it was crazy.

Community nurses are fundamental to general practice and the broader primary care. They provide invaluable services, particularly for the very young, older and infirm patients, and those with severe mental illness. Sadly, the latter two particularly are just the groups that have little leverage on public policy. Community nurses are highly trained specialists in their fields, and helpful to GPs for both their clinical work and professional advice. In my experience, that advice was always given in a friendly, non-judgemental manner, effectively concealing the nurse's amazement that I needed to ask the question in the first place.

The community nursing professions receive too little recognition. We, and more importantly our patients, would have been lost without our midwife, health visitors, district nurses, and community psychiatric nurses. Is this lack of recognition, this invisibility until we need them, in part because their work is intentionally peripatetic? GPs have their surgeries with out-of-date magazines and posters; dentists have their practices, pictures on the ceiling, and whirring drills; specialists have their hospitals with long corridors; and opticians their high-street premises with trendy glasses in the window. We can picture any of them.

But community nurses are, well, wherever they are. They are intangible. That they come to our homes is part of their strength and value. They are the greatest domiciliary component of the NHS, particularly since the virtual demise of GP visits.

With the movement of services away from hospitals and back into the community, their stars are surely in the ascendancy. They must be so. They are vital members of many peoples' Myteam, and will be ever more important members of the PHCT.

***

A useful economic guideline in medicine is that you should only do what only you can do. In the past, at least, GPs were most certainly in breach of that principle, and always had been. What were we doing filling out forms for investigations by hand, taking blood samples during consultations, or seeing patients for routine antenatal appointments or regular checks of their well-controlled hypertension? Every one of those would be done better and with a greater overall economy by someone else. Equally, the blood samples should not be delegated to nurses – they also have duties that only they are trained to do. A phlebotomist is trained to take blood samples.

That is just the sort of fragmentation of general practice described by Professor Spurgeon in the chapter titled "Information Systems: the Paper Years". At a human level it may be regrettable, but here I believe the economic argument holds sway.

Practice nurses differ from community nurses by being employed directly by the practice and by usually working within the practice building. Their forte is preventive medicine and chronic disease management, though they may well also attend to the straightforward elements of acute care. Their work is of incalculable value to the modern practice, leaving the doctors to do what only they can do: generalised diagnostics and therapeutics, and the rapid, simultaneous consideration of multiple problems. Some say others could do these tasks. Of course, with suitable training they could indeed; but then they would be a GP.

I long maintained that there was a need for more nurses in general practice. We were among the first to climb above a ratio of 1:1 to doctors, but that was still far below the 2.5:1 ration I had seen in a Kaiser Permanente centre in Los Angeles. Within any healthcare system, the cost of doctors should preclude them from doing anything that others can also do, let alone doing it better.

Here is a clear illustration that the overall clinical task of the practice can be achieved more efficiently with appropriate sharing of the work between appropriately skilled clinicians. Patient care is different from the past, less personal no doubt, but unarguably better for such teamwork.

MAKING IT HAPPEN: MANAGING A PRACTICE

Management is doing things right. Leadership is doing the right things.

Peter F Drucker

In the late 1970s, the potential of NHS general practice began to be realised through the evolving interest of GPs in actively managing their work. After all, these were medium-sized businesses with responsibilities not only for themselves and their thousands of patients but also for disbursing, directly or indirectly, very substantial sums of public money. As with the uptake of most innovations, first came the early adopters with their playful curiosity, but it required a mighty, contractual kick for there to be universal uptake. This chapter discusses the evolution of management within practices.

THE DEVELOPMENT OF PRACTICE MANAGEMENT

Before the 1980s, the organisation within most practices consisted of filing patients' records in alphabetical order and keeping the accountancy books. Consultations usually took place in the doctor's home, the patient's home, or in small, unconverted commercial premises. There were no staff other than part-time receptionists and the doctors' wives, and patients themselves usually initiated contacts between a doctor and themselves.

The contract that followed the 1965 Charter facilitated change that gathered pace in the 1970s, not least by reimbursing 70% of the cost of ancillary staff up to a limit of 2 per doctor. Indirectly, this also encouraged group practice, because the crude calculation meant each additional doctor permitted the disproportionate employment of two more heavily subsidised staff. Embryonic PHCTs began to develop, echoing early pioneers and working from converted premises or purpose-designed medical and health centres. GPs were mostly free from accountability and in broad terms could define their tasks under an umbrella of considerable job security.

Of course, the profession had its visionary prophets. John Fry, an eminent and remarkable pioneer of modern practice, wrote in 1965 that he felt the most important need was to inculcate self-enquiry and self-checking into doctors, to teach them to examine and analyse their work so that they could seek to improve the work of their practices.

He collected information from his daily activities on simple card systems, examined that information, and then used the results for self-education, practice management, and for writing groundbreaking research papers and textbooks on the content of general practice.

His workload was prodigious, to the point that many felt he must be using assistants and other helpers. He did not. As a trainee, I was fascinated by his whole approach and went to visit him. What struck me was his ability to perform the ultimate clinical trick of combining effortless efficiency with a relaxed and apparently unhurried manner with patients. He was an inspiration to me and I based my manual workload analysis system on his card index.

Another pioneer was Geoff Marsh, a GP in Stockton-on-Tees and an enthusiast for, among many other things, the efficient deployment of staff.[148]

Even earlier, between the two world wars, Dr W Pickles was recording epidemiological studies within his country practice in

---

[148] Marsh GN (1967). Group practice nurse: an analysis and comment on six months' work. *Bri Med J*, 1(5538): 489–491.

Wensleydale, Yorkshire. Apart from many published articles he wrote one of the classics of epidemiological research.[149]

He combined groundbreaking research with compassionate devotion to his patients and is considered one of the all-time giants of general practice. During a lecture, he described his thoughts on looking down on Wensleydale from a hilltop:

> *One by one I made out most of our grey villages with their thin pall of smoke. And as I watched the evening train creeping up the valley with its pauses at our three stations, a quaint thought came into my head and it was that there was hardly a man, woman or child in all those villages of whom I did not know the Christian name and with whom I was not on terms of intimate friendship. My wife and I say that we know most of the dogs and, indeed some of the cats.[150]*

It was not until the 1990 contract that GP training included the acquisition of management skills. Previously, there had been a nonchalant feeling within the hierarchy of the profession that management was a matter of common sense. The influential book *The Future General Practitioner: Teaching and Learning*, published by the RCGP in 1972, began its chapter on practice management with:

> *It might be said that this chapter is unnecessary; if there is one subject with which teachers should be comfortable and familiar it is practice organisation, especially their own.*

To be fair, the book implied a rather narrow use of the word, referring to managing personnel within larger practices. Yet, the greatest benefits would be the ability of doctors to manage themselves, set objectives for the practice, plan how to achieve them, and review progress and results. These were the very things that John Fry had

---

[149] Pickles WN (1939). *Epidemiology in Country Practice*. Bristol, Wright.
[150] Moorhead R (2001). Pickles of Wensleydale. *J R Soc Med*, 94(10): 536–540.

called for in 1965 and which appear to have been ignored seven years later by the working group that wrote *The Future General Practitioner*.

I have still not found a better and more succinct summary of the need for clear and concise management than that written in 1969 for the Industrial Society by Margaret Brown:

> *It is essential that an organisation asks – and answers – two vital questions: 'what do we exist for?', and 'what key activities do we need to do outstandingly well?' A formal structure must then be designed to make possible the attainment of these objectives and the successful performance of the key activities.*[151]

I think she would have got on very well with John Fry.

Dr McGuinness was the first to suggest that practices might construct an annual report identifying their objectives and results.[152] He was a senior lecturer at Liverpool University and with three colleagues had set up a new practice in Runcorn, Cheshire. They began writing annual reports in 1977, but there were no textbooks on the subject until 1984.[153]

By the mid-1980s, things were starting to pick up. Although the college had published its Quality Initiative,[154] the word "management" was still seen by many GPs as inappropriate to their work when used in the context of practice administration. For them, it had unsavoury overtones of business and making money. (Perversely, it was – and still is – used commonly in a clinical context, such as in "the

---

[151] Brown M (1969). *The Manager's Guide to the Behavioural Sciences. Notes for Managers Series.* London, Industrial Society.

[152] McGuiness BW (1980). Why not a practice annual report? *J R Coll Gen Pract*, 30(221): 744.

[153] Pritchard PMM, Low K, Whalen M (1984). *Management in General Practice.* Oxford, OUP.

[154] Irvine DH (1983). Quality of care in general practice: our outstanding problem. *J R Coll Gen Pract*, 33: 521–523.

management of diabetes".) The definition used in this chapter comes from the *International Dictionary of Management*,[155] though it would do pretty well as a definition of clinical management also:

> *The effective utilisation and coordination of resources such as capital, plant, materials and labour to achieve defined objectives with maximum efficiency.*

The need for such management in general practice was all too apparent. There were greater demands on the resources available than could be met in full. Given such scarcity, there was a responsibility to use resources efficiently, for in the grand order of things one task inevitably involved a sacrifice somewhere else. Nor was the situation the same in hospitals, where there were management structures designed to coordinate all aspects of the administration. Within general practice, with its fiercely defended independent contractor status, GPs themselves had to ensure the optimal deployment of the available resources. Such consideration was not just about the patient in question, but also the service to the entire practice population and, as I have already discussed, populations beyond also.

***

MANAGEMENT TRAINING: IF ALL ELSE FAILS, DO IT YOURSELF

In the late-1970s, our neighbour was a Danish architect on the construction team of Northampton's Carlsberg brewery. One day, he showed me his time management system, a structured system rather like a Filofax on anabolic steroids. He told me the Danish company

---

[155] Johannsen H, Page GT (2002). *International Dictionary of Management.* New Delhi, Crest Publishing House.

Time Management International ran management training courses in London, and suggested I went on one.

The course cost £90 for the day at the Hotel Café Royal in Regent Street. I approached the education authorities at Oxford RHA only to be told, of course, that this would be unsuitable for funding as it was a management course.

I went in any case, and it was fantastic, the most valuable single day of postgraduate training I ever had. Around the table, I joined executives from companies such as Shell, BMW, Rank Xerox, and IBM. The company had never had a doctor on a course before, so staff and delegates were all inquisitive about this meddlesome medic within their managerial midst.

"What, objectively, does your job entail?" they enquired. I was not sure. The astonishing, official "A GP does what GPs do" did not sound very objective to me, and I kept that gem from my executive classmates.

"Even if you did know what you were trying to do" joined in my polite but ruthless course tutors, "how would you know whether or not you were doing it?"

"Are you doing your job this year better than last year, or worse, or do you not care?"

"How would you like your practice to develop over the next year, and over the next 10 years?"

Oh dear. This was not going well at all. I felt embarrassed. It had terrible echoes of my anatomy training with the heron-like professor, back at medical school. Worse, while the level of anatomical detail required at medical school was absurd (and is no longer needed), these questions were the very alphabet of organisation and management, and clearly I was illiterate. I should know the answers, but did not have a clue.

Very few practices addressed such questions at that time, for GPs had little incentive to improve the services they offered other than altruism, a notoriously unreliable motivating factor. Audits that would have been considered matters of regular routine management review in any successful small business, or for that matter in many unsuccessful ones, were dressed up and published in our journals as original research. The problem was exactly that. They were not routine; they were so novel, so new, that in our world they were indeed research.

Meanwhile, we were attempting to undertake the task that was in its totality beyond us. That is inherent in a comprehensive, open access system with a finite budget. Practices must, therefore, identify the work to be done and their priorities, establish the resources available to them, use those resources as wisely as possible in undertaking the work, and check they are doing what they think they are doing. Plan, acquire resources, do, review – we might think of this as the four-point model for doing absolutely anything.[156] The cycle describes common sense; we all use it every day, whether going shopping, planning and enjoying a summer holiday, performing open heart surgery, or landing a man on the moon.

Back at the Hotel Café Royal, despite my embarrassment, I knew those were exactly the type of questions I wanted to be able to address. Incredibly, by the end of the day, I had a plan, a structure, for doing general practice as I wanted to do it. I used it for the next 30 years and even now it is one I would not change. It is no coincidence that it forms the basic structure of this book.

***

Occasionally, over the years we obtained external management advice. In the late 1970s, we were part of a research project within the Oxford Region, in which senior managers from industry were

---

[156] Its common title is the Plan, Do, Review Cycle, but there is value in adding the fourth element of resource acquisition, particularly in the circumstances we are considering here.

contracted to work a few sessions with individual practices. Cliff Woods was the personnel director of a major UK company. He had never worked with a practice before; perhaps the exercise was across waters as uncharted for him as they were for us.

For the first time, all those working within the practice – doctors, receptionists, and attached nurses – sat down and considered what we were trying to do, and how we were doing it. I remember our initial incredulity, even hostility, that he thought we might not know such things already, and that someone from outside had the temerity to come in and ask us such questions. I remember his charm and skill in coaxing us to a gradual realisation that we did not know after all, and that the exercise was useful. I also remember his comment at the end that he had never come across such a complex team structure in all his years in personnel management. What struck him about our practice was the mix of different clinical disciplines, employers, employees, and responsibilities within such a small group. The role of every single person was unique and necessary for our success.

PANNELL KERR FORSTER

Our most productive dalliance with management expertise came in 1991–1992 when our practice manager, Julie Trew, unearthed the business planning initiative for small businesses operated by the DTI. The deal was that if we paid 50% of the costs, we would be allocated 15 full days of a consultant's time. The DTI would cover the organisation and everything else. Our consultant was Simon Oldfield from Pannell Kerr Forster, one of the world's largest accountancy firms, and the task we agreed with him was to develop a management structure and business plan. Our first 5 days were in November 1991, with the final 10 the following July. At the time we did not realise how pivotal the exercise was to the future of the practice.

The practice now consisted of a list of 8000.[157] There were 5 partners (3 full-time, 2 part-time) supported by 19 reception, office, and nursing staff. Our overall task and mission, in management-speak, was to be "committed to developing a thriving practice which provides the best personal, primary medical care possible given the available resources." Simon's initial, detailed business analysis identified four key areas for action.

First, personnel. Michael Woolmore was due to retire in two years, and Simon encouraged us to start planning for that. Team role analysis showed four of the five partners saw themselves as ideas people and resource investigators. "The overall implication is that the practice creates many ideas and is very innovative in its approach. However, the failing is a lack of follow-through to ensure that ideas are practical, cost-effective, and working as originally intended." Prescient words indeed.

Second, premises. No matter how lovely it was, we had outgrown our extended building in Billing Road. We needed "to move to new premises more suited to the demands placed upon today's general medical practitioner."

Third, management. We would do better through structured monthly meetings, having more time to discuss key issues, and obtaining better harnessing of skills.

Fourth, information. He encouraged us to move away from time-consuming, experimental computer systems to ones which simply did what we most wanted.

So, what happened? Two years after the DTI project, we were in a new purpose-built building. We had withdrawn from much of our experimental computer work and moved from VAMP to EMIS, a computer system that allowed us to consult without paper records. There was a carefully planned structure of strategic clinical team and

---

[157] We had recently deliberately reduced the list to try to manage an increasing workload.

administrative meetings for different groups within the practice, and we had a replacement partner safely installed. And we had a large car park.

Why did that project make a difference, enabling such profound changes? First, Simon came with credibility; we respected his skills and were inclined to follow his lead. His interpersonal skills were excellent and his analyses spot on, even though we might not have always liked them. Second, he managed us brilliantly, helping us to look critically and dispassionately at what we were trying to do and what changes were required if we were to do it. The exercise was not just a talking shop; he helped us achieve very real results.

FINDING OUT WHAT PATIENTS THOUGHT

At the beginning of 1994, our thoughts turned to the matter of finding what our patients thought about the services we were providing. Of course, we got a subjective impression from day-to-day contacts, but a problem here is that most patients do not like upsetting their doctors, particularly those they know well. So, if we just asked them, face-to-face, we received a very slanted reply, which was almost invariably positive. That was not the basis for planning how to alter things. It is nice to know what is good, but more useful to know what is not.

Here we made further use of home-grown children. My son Paul needed a project for his psychology degree at City University, London. He was interested in undertaking a satisfaction survey among our patients. Having a service satisfaction survey, and one constructed with supervised academic rigour was very useful and gave us the opportunity to repeat it for comparison. We did that in June 1995, using his brother Mark, and again in July 1997 using our new patient liaison officer. On both occasions, we used samples of the same size, and age and sex distribution, as in 1994 and obtained very similar response rates.

The results showed that in general, patients were most pleased with matters concerning interpersonal skills, such as feeling welcome in the practice and not being made to feel they were a nuisance or wasting time. They were less happy with what the survey termed impersonal matters, such as getting through to the surgery on the phone, and delays waiting to be seen once inside the building.

Perhaps the most pleasing high score was for the statement: "When I enter the practice I feel very welcome." The statement receiving the worst negative score of all was: "I am always able to arrange an appointment for exactly when I want one." Some things never change. In the subsequent repeat surveys both the impersonal and interpersonal scores improved year on year, though as in 1994, the impersonal dimension lagged behind.

After 1997, we stopped repeating the survey because new regulations required all practices to use a nationally organised survey each year. Better through uniformity, perhaps, but here was another nail in the coffin of innovation.

THE MILLENNIUM

If we now jump forward to 2000, we can see several significant changes in the management of the practice. The partnership had increased to five whole time equivalents, and the list of patients had increased by 6% in the year. There was an increasing emphasis on the work of practice nurses in preventive care and chronic disease management, typically within clinics using the practice's protocols and computer templates.

There was an annual cycle of clinical audits, with monthly meetings rotating through ischaemic heart disease, diabetes, asthma and chronic obstructive pulmonary disease (COPD), epilepsy, thyroid disease, repeat prescribing, referrals, strokes, deaths, hypertension, workload, and smoking cessation. For each meeting, Carole Hyde, our clinical governance and information manager, undertook the analyses and reporting.

We had developed a continuing professional development programme with half-day meetings taking place twice a month, one with a clinical agenda and a parallel one for administrative staff. And the practice had established a significant event review system that ensured the constructive debate of possible clinical and administrative errors. All told, this was a structure that might well have pleased my course at the Hotel Café Royal two decades earlier.

***

Finally, in this chapter, I will include an excerpt from the *Contact* newsletter of our PSG. This group provided a valuable opinion about the future direction of the practice and current services. They also raised funds to help buy additional facilities for patients and represented the practice in local and national patient group meetings.

Perhaps their greatest contribution, however, was the excellent quarterly newsletter they distributed to our patients, both within the building and also, notably, posted out free to all those flagged on our systems as being housebound.

Issue 45 came out in March 2004 and contained an article from the practice about the new contract due to come into force the following month. Again, it offers an insight into our thinking at the time:

> *In April 2004 a new contract will come into operation for all NHS general practices. Most changes will be organisational rather than dramatically different. Patients will register with the practice rather than an individual doctor and although GPs can now opt out of doing night work, when the surgery is closed NORMED[158] will continue just as now.*

---

[158] NORMED was the existing out of hours service run by Northampton's GPs.

Change usually brings disadvantages as well as benefits. What, on balance, will be the effect for patients and the King Edward Road surgery?[159] Will the latest set of changes win the prize of making NHS general practice as good as it should be, or will it be more like British tennis players, providing more hope than realistic expectation?[160]

The emphasis of the contract is on improving the quality of care given to patients. Good; no one could argue with that. But that means more counting and measurement so that health authorities and the DoH know whether things are getting better. So, we will inevitably spend more time putting information into computers during consultations. Not so good.

It also means there will be less flexibility; we will have to follow the rules and regulations more rigidly. For example, we will have no choice but to ensure that patients have a review of long-term medication. Better care perhaps, but less consideration for the wishes of the individual patient. There will be more opportunities for you to let us know what you think, increasing the role of our PSG. We will be learning from a regular, annual survey of patients and opinions about our services. Finding out what patients think is a good thing.

The effect of the new contract will be that we have more information about the services we provide regarding our preventive medicine programme, acute care service, and the increasingly important follow-up of ongoing conditions. If the NHS can do that as a whole, to a high standard, it will indeed do something very special. The new contract plays its part by making a genuine advance in the quality of care provided by general practices. But it is not the runaway victory that politicians would like you to believe.

***

---

[159] Our half of the Christchurch Medical Centre.

[160] Clearly, this remark was made before the ascent of Andy Murray, who at the time was only a teenager, and is ranked number 1 by the Association of Tennis Professionals at the time of writing this book.

Over the remaining couple of years of my career, the practice undertook two further management exercises, but I will reserve them for the chapter titled "Putting It All into Practice".

PART FIVE

POLITICAL FORCES

The NHS is one of the most potent, dominant political forces in the UK. For economic, ideological, and political reasons, every new government wants to alter it. A particularly challenging set of changes took place in the early 1990s, and Part Five uses these as an example of the opposing forces and political intrigue involved.

As in Part Four, it also demonstrates how determined, freethinking, independent GPs can make innovative and important advances in local and national health services, particularly when they work together.

WORKING WITH THE AUTHORITIES

It is amazing what you can accomplish if you do not care who gets the credit.

Harry S Truman

In 1990, Margaret Thatcher's government introduced the NHS internal market – the most profound change in the service since its inception and one that has grown in importance ever since.[161] For the first time, a division would be created between those providing NHS services and those requiring – and therefore purchasing – them.

Now gamekeepers were to turn poachers. Far from the health authorities managing the local hospitals, as had happened in the past, now they were to buy services from them, or indeed any other hospital, within a competitive market.

But health authorities were not the only purchasers. If they wished, GPs could apply to hold a budget (or fund, as the government quickly learnt to call it, as budget too clearly indicated its intention) with which they could buy a relatively small but significant range of hospital services on behalf of their patients. Initially, the largest purchasers by far were the health authorities, which purchased all the services required for non-fundholding practices and 80% of those for fundholders. Nonetheless, fundholding was a foot in the door, a bold initiative. Practices had the option whether or not to become

---

[161] HM Government (1989). *Working for Patients*. London, HMSO.

fundholders, but that was clearly the direction of government policy. Initially, the scheme was a small snowball on a large downhill slope, but one with friends in high places to push it and the potential to grow enormous.

Much has been written about GP fundholding, but less about its main alternative, locality commissioning, which was invented by GPs and health authorities in response to the market. That is why I describe an example here, the one in Northampton of which I have experience. Of course, I take a position on the internal market. That is what a market does. It divides us; it forces choice.

***

JOB CREATION

When the changes were first announced, one thing quickly became apparent. If the authorities were to be effective purchasers, they needed GPs to work jointly with them. I found this idea appealing. There was scope for creativity, and if you felt the reforms were misguided, as I did, then it was incumbent on you to come up with better ideas. I arranged to reduce my commitment in the practice and to work half time as liaison GP for Northampton Health Authority. My job was to bridge the impending divide between hospitals, the health authority, fundholders, non-fundholders, and the Northamptonshire FHSA.[162]

THE NORTHAMPTON EXPERIENCE

At the end of 1989, the district's GPs already felt the winds of impending change and formed a core group to represent them

---

[162] FHSAs had taken over the control and oversight of the four branches of primary care. As such, they were responsible for supervising local fundholders, though RHAs selected the practices.

concerning hospital services. Faced with the future market economy, the core group developed a Statement of Priorities on 22 January 1991. Its interest in local cohesion was evident in the wording of the introduction:

> *In setting out our priorities, the group is only too aware of the difficulties experienced by the hospital. We see the process of implementing the April 1st NHS changes as a two-way exercise in which GPs should expect to play their part. A continuing limitation of resources is an inevitability that all clinicians must accept, no matter how sadly. These statements of priorities assume an atmosphere of cooperation in which GPs strive to improve the effectiveness of their use of hospital services while the hospital departments themselves seek ways to meet, amongst other things, the priorities of GPs.*

That statement chimed with my own thinking and with that of most people in the health authority, and it would underpin our joint approach.

Well before the starting gun for the reforms on 1 April 1991 was fired, the core group decided to work on the one hand with the health authority about planning services, and on the other with senior hospital staff about issues relating to clinical management. Over the following years, it proved an effective, two-part strategy.

The previous year, the core group had conceived specialty liaison groups (SLGs) as a common sense means of encouraging specialists and GPs to work together.[163] Their task was to find ways of making the best use of the resources available for a particular speciality or condition. They functioned as small, informal groups of two or three GPs, a similar number of consultants from the relevant speciality, and a plate of sandwiches. They agreed on simple objectives based on the problems of each side, and then decided methods of addressing them

---

[163] Willis A (1997). Speciality liaison groups. In: *Professional Development in General Practice*. Pendleton D and Hasler J (eds). Oxford, OUP, pp. 134–147.

within the existing resource allocation. That was a ground rule set by the core group to prevent hospital departments using the groups as a means to inveigle additional funds out of the health authority.

Every SLG contained a member of the core group, which could take up relevant matters within its regular meetings with the health authority, though usually this was just as a courtesy. Most of Northampton's clinicians did not like the idea of the internal market and turned with relief to SLGs as a means of improving quality and efficiency without having to get involved in divisive buying and selling.

We started with six SLGs, but by the end of 1992 that number had risen to 32 and covered all the main speciality departments as well as specific clinical areas, such as epilepsy, heart failure, radiology, and asthma. After the initial six, it was the specialists who proposed them all. SLGs simply made sense to everyone. If there were 150 GPs in the district and only two consultants in a speciality, then both groups realised they should get together and work out how best to make use of that specialist resource. During 1992 alone, over 100 clinicians were directly involved in the 32 SLGs, some in more than one.

***

The other limb of the strategy raised the question of how practices were to engage in the internal market. This was vexatious for a whole variety of practical, philosophical, and reactionary reasons. The GP core group came up with the idea of running a project to evaluate the different options available. Again the task was simple: to find the best way to improve local health services for patients in a manner consistent with the guiding principles of the NHS and within the context of the government's 1990 NHS Reforms. If some saw the project as politically partisan, that was because it had the temerity to evaluate, let alone challenge, the government's prevailing dogma. To think it primarily a political exercise was to afford party politics a higher status in our minds than they deserved.

The Options in Purchasing (OIP) project was formally established in June 1992 and funded jointly by the DHA and FHSA. As liaison GP, I was asked to lead it, and as our independent external adviser we employed Professor Chris Ham from the Health Services Management Centre, University of Birmingham.[164] As we anticipated, it was his involvement that gave our project much-needed gravitas within the circles of power. There were already three fundholding practices in the health district, but the primary purpose was to inform the 43 non-fundholding practices about the opportunities available to them.

The project team considered all the options available, from complete head-in-the-sand denial of the internal market, through working with the health authority as our sole purchaser, individual fundholding, and the development of a coordinated "superfund".[165] We also invented our own, additional option.

In late 1992, we reported to a meeting of the district's GPs, recommending the development of what we called "locality commissioning with central purchasing". (A few weeks later, I was pleasantly surprised to receive a phone call from the British Library asking if they could have a copy of the report for their "archives of important documents".[166] Sadly, neither the government nor the DoH made such a request.)

The report and its strategy were accepted by the division of GPs. Within the next few days, all 14 of the local practices that had applied for the second wave of fundholding withdrew their applications,

---

[164] Chris Ham was Professor of Health Policy and Management at the University of Birmingham. In April 2010, he became Chief Executive of the King's Fund in London.
[165] Here everybody would become a fundholder and pool their funds to work together.
[166] Northampton Health Authority (1992). *Northampton Options in Purchasing Project: Final Report, Phase B*. British Library Catalogue ref: OP-LG/7445.

individually; they preferred to go with the district's plan. We had not been aware of their applications and only heard of their withdrawal later from a furious RHA, which never forgave us. In itself that says much about the pressure put on GPs to become fundholders, particularly within the Oxford Region.

We felt the district's commissioning should be based on three localities to increase its sensitivity to local needs while retaining populations large enough for significant needs assessment and risk sharing. However, we felt that procurement should remain with the statutory health authority. Whereas we saw commissioning as planning what needed doing, we considered procurement as buying the required services to fulfil those plans. This arrangement reflected the concerns of many doctors about ethics and equity while providing economies of scale regarding population size, expertise, and administrative endeavour.

An interesting detail was that the project recommended the use, where appropriate, of practice-specific contracts. The health authority would place a contract with a hospital outside the district for the specific use of a practice that had good reason to use the services of such a hospital. For example, it might well be more convenient for patients living on the edge of our geographical district to go to a hospital close to them, but across the boundary in another health district. This was a breathtakingly simple way of increasing the sensitivity of contracts to the needs of local communities. They offered similar contracting flexibility to the fundholding scheme, but with the added benefits of centralised, coordinated purchasing and the potential to cover the full 100% of services provided, rather than the 20% achievable by a fundholder.

One of the most interesting options considered by the OIP was for all of us to become fundholders and pool our resources into one large, district-wide superfund. We would then manage the fund's 20% of services while working closely with the health authority, particularly about the 80% of services it would still purchase on our behalf. The arrangement would maintain the local cohesion we felt so important and reduce the chance of some patients getting priority over others for financial reasons. It would provide all our practices with the additional resources made available to fundholders, and yet benefit from economies of scale and pooled expertise. And it would be very close indeed to what the government was pressing us to do in any case. The idea had a lot of merit for everyone.

However, it was rejected at the exploratory stage by the Oxford RHA. As the OIP project manager, I had phoned the RHA to discuss the idea. Rather than being overjoyed by our approach, the senior manager I spoke to seemed thoroughly alarmed. They would not allow it. They would be unable to cope with managing the 32 funds we were proposing for our 47 practices.[167] And neither, he said, would our FHSA be able to administer so many funds. This was an intriguing observation given it was the logical end point of national policy.

Leaving that aside, he missed an opportunity. If he had run with our idea, he would have had a unified, district-wide GP commissioning and purchasing project that worked closely with its health authority. It would be several years before the government rolled out the same idea as large-scale pilots of what it termed "total purchasing". Oxford would have achieved the nationwide acclaim it so obviously craved. Even further ahead, our scheme would, in organisational terms, have looked remarkably like the present CCGs.

In any case, we developed an alternative option, one that we felt was better, and one that eventually helped form a future government's NHS policy. That manager's blinkered, unthinking reaction may have wasted several years. In truth, we might well have gone with the

---

[167] The regulations decreed that small practices would have to join others for fundholding. Here, at least, we see a glancing concern for the economic dangers of small populations.

option we selected in any case. We will never know; the district-wide superfund was no longer an option.

What we do know is that our preferred solution was far cheaper. Had we been allowed to set up 32 funds in a 42-practice superfund, the set-up allowances alone paid to the practices by the NHS would have run to approximately £1.5 million. Ongoing practice administrative allowances would have come to about £1 million per year at 1992 prices.

In comparison, locality commissioning with central purchasing attracted no additional funding at all. It seems reasonable to conclude that in 1992–1993, the practices in the Northampton District "saved" the NHS about £2.5 million on administrative and computer allowances alone by not becoming fundholders. Unfortunately, that saving was not available to develop local services. Another way of looking at those figures is that they represent the money that government policy was in large part depriving the non-fundholders of in our district. Nonetheless, I believe our approach created at least as much beneficial change as we would have achieved as single-practice fundholders. Meanwhile, we retained equity and local cooperation between specialists, GPs, and managers, and saved £2.5 million for the Exchequer in our first year.

TAKING IT A STEP FURTHER

Some of us within the health authority were keen to expand the concept of locality commissioning, recognising the need to involve a broader group of agencies than only the GPs and health authority in the process. A project was commissioned and funded by the FHSA, the two health authorities in the county, and the Department of Social Services (now largely replaced by the Department for Work & Pensions), its objective being to establish a means for interagency collaboration at a locality level. An external consultant, David Webster, and I were asked to undertake the work.

Here was an effort to engage everyone – all primary care professions allied to medicine, such as physiotherapy and chiropody, hospital services, the voluntary sector, local government, the public, and social services – to work together to improve care in its broadest sense. To say it was ambitious would be an understatement.

Our report, *A Sense of Place*,[168] promoted a new body, the interagency locality team, whose task would be to bring together all those different parties, and for these parties to work in a cohesive manner. The report contained a model that embraced their differing requirements while minimising bureaucracy. It was locality commissioning taken to its logical conclusion. Looking back, its breadth of local cooperation now appears very like the arrangements within the 2011 Bill for creating a local joint strategic needs assessment and strategy.

A Sense of Place also recognised that the concept of locality commissioning, with central purchasing confined to hospital services, might well prove merely a transitional stage. It suggested that some form of pooled budget would eventually be required to fully engage interagency locality teams, to break down the silo mentality of the different agencies, instil a sense of financial reality, and encourage everyone to work together, with major cost and service benefits. Of course, the task of establishing such a budget, gleaned from the sparse resources of agencies such as health and social services, would be highly problematic for a host of reasons.

***

For all its unpopularity with the RHA and the DoH, our Northampton system worked. A survey of all our GPs in December 1993 (response rate of 85%) found that almost 80% of

---

[168] Willis A (2017). *The Practice Matters Archive*. [online] Available from http://practice-matters.co.uk/index.php/the-practice-matters-archive/ (accessed 9 January 2017).

respondents either agreed or strongly agreed that they were influencing purchasing decisions through the Northampton approach. We did not decry the voluntary fundholding scheme, and we were not "antifundholding", as many of our critics claimed. Indeed, our fundholders were included and, as it happens, by their scarcity inevitably overrepresented in the core and locality groups.

Our approach recognised that those who wished to become fundholders should do so, but that it was a voluntary scheme and opportunities should be developed for non-fundholders to contribute equally to the evolution of local services on behalf of their patients. Within our health district, we wanted equity of access for patients, beneficial cooperation between hospitals and GPs, and equality of opportunity for practices. National policy deliberately denied those principles, leaving us with no choice but to invent a different way to develop our local health service; in our eyes a better way. It seems fair to say the next government agreed with us.

REFORMING THE REFORMS

If the government's ideas for involving GPs in the internal market were fundamentally flawed, as many believed, what could be done about it? It was no use sitting on one's hands and just shouting abuse from the sidelines. Nationally, we had to come up with better ideas, and preferably ones acceptable to the government.

First, many fundholders improved the situation dramatically by coalescing into multifunds to gain from economies of scale. Second, non-fundholders developed LCGs and ways of working closely with their health authorities. Different approaches, but with similar effects. Both harnessed the inventive abilities of GPs to create new ways of working, using the differing resources and opportunities available to them. In earlier chapters, we saw this entrepreneurial flare of GPs at a practice level, concerning the development of buildings, staff, and information systems.

* * *

In Northampton, we were aware that other places were exploring similar alternatives to our own; we had visited several during the OIP project. But we did not know their extent. No one did. These were subversive activities; few heath authorities would proclaim them for fear of direct or indirect reprisals from the DoH.

That is not being overdramatic. Nationally, I know it was made clear to some senior staff at health authorities and FHSAs that there was a risk to their jobs if they did not promote and deliver fundholding, but rather supported alternative approaches such as GP commissioning. Yet, as I have already explained, fundholding was a choice for GPs, an optional approach for their engagement with the internal market. A stated alternative option, according to the government and DoH, was for them to work with their health authority, yet this was vigorously undermined and discouraged in a variety of ways. The duplicity of politicians and civil servants was as astonishing as it was disappointing. Journalists and even some economists were in thrall to the positive publicity surrounding fundholding.

In fact, in Northampton, we were by no means alone in our activities, and this section describes how different groups from far and wide coalesced to form a national movement of real influence.

***

Alan Birchall was a GP in Nottingham. Along with three colleagues, he wrote a letter to the *BMJ* in 1994 saying he was involved in a group of non-fundholding practices working with their health authority. The letter asked if any like-minded GPs would be interested in setting up or joining a national association.[169] He received dozens of replies from all over the UK. Here was Darwinian convergent evolution: different pockets of innovation were arising, isolated from each other by a lack of communication, yet developing in similar ways. One such example was in Telford, Shropshire, where the chair was Dr Quentin Shaw. The Telford group was already thinking of organising a national meeting for similar groups. Quentin got in touch with Alan and, encouraged by the number of responses to the letter, organised a conference.

Forty-six people attended the meeting on 12 March 1994, including non-fundholders, managers, academics, and a few fundholders. It was remarkable for its bonhomie, its confluence of like minds, and its quiet, collective resolve to do something at a national level. A temporary committee of five was selected to meet in the near

---

[169] Black DG, Trimble IM, Birchall AD, et al. (1994). General practice fundholding. Non-fundholding groups better for everyone. *BMJ*, 308(6926): 476–477.

future to set up a national organisation. A few weeks later, the committee met, for geographical convenience in the lounge of Northampton's Swallow Hotel, just off the M1 motorway and in the middle of the country. Provided we bought occasional cups of coffee, the staff seemed perfectly happy for us to sit in a corner for a couple of hours and plan great things. The hotel has changed its name now, but it is still the same building, with its function inevitably developed over time. And the same can be said for the plans we made that day. No longer the same name, but they also evolved, eventually contributing DNA to PCGs and from there the current CCGs. It must have been strong coffee.

We agreed on a temporary executive structure and a name, the National Association of Commissioning GPs (NACGP), sticking to the view that the word included planning and review, but excluded purchasing. An apt logo seemed to be an image of Telford's Ironbridge, the site of our first meeting and also the birthplace of the Industrial Revolution, and we adopted the slogan "bridging the divide".

That said it all. Our intention was to bridge the divides appearing between fundholders and non-fundholders, specialists and generalists, hospitals and health authorities. We wanted to bring together everyone who had a part to play in the development of local health services, to ensure that any changes were beneficial within the philosophical framework of the NHS. And ours was indeed a revolution; we were seeking better ways than existed already. Again, we were neither critical of our fundholding colleagues nor against them, but we wanted everyone included in bringing about beneficial change, whether they chose to be fundholders or not.

The NACGP was an exciting organisation. In the beginning, it had no money and was not even recognised by the doctrinaire Secretary of State for Health, Virginia Bottomley. Our efforts to help improve the NHS through locality commissioning were not encouraged;

frequently, they were maliciously undermined. We were not toeing the party line. Inevitably, the guns of the political thought police were turned on us.

It was all rather exhilarating. We knew our case was unanswerable. An unfettered market operating at single-practice level contradicted the fundamental principles of the NHS, notably the right of patients to be treated equitably, according to their relative need. What we were up against were the powerful, vested interests of politicians and NHS policymakers, who had the misfortune to have created, and then backed, a congenitally flawed horse. Fortunately, with careful breeding mainly bioengineered by GP fundholders themselves, that original bloodline quickly improved.

Despite all the undermining of our efforts and successes, most GPs liked our ideas. In January 1995, a survey in *Pulse*, a GP newspaper usually hostile to locality commissioning, found that 75% of GPs would vote to abolish fundholding and the internal market. Presciently, almost exactly half thought the reforms meant GPs, rather than the government, would take the blame for rationing within the NHS. I am surprised the figure was that low.

By the time of the next general election, in May 1997, another GP newspaper poll found that 75% of respondents favoured locality commissioning as a model for future primary care involvement. This was a remarkable result given that by then half of GPs were fundholders of one form or another. (Though how many respondents were fundholders, it is not known.) As Ron Singer later said:

> *NACGP is an outstanding example of ordinary people having an unfashionable idea and bringing it to national and international attention, against the odds.*[170]

---

[170] Singer R (ed.) (1997). *GP Commissioning: an Inevitable Evolution.* Abingdon, Radcliffe Medical Press, p. 17. This book is the definitive account of the original GP commissioning movement.

The active core of the NACGP was tiny. At a national level, it was its 10-strong executive committee, and we were spread all over the country. We had no premises or staff, almost no money, only our spare time to work in, and an obsession with frugality even George Osborne would admire. In 1995, the total expenditure for running this national association for a year was just £460.

And yet, we had to look big to carry any weight, and such illusion was the key to our credibility. Over the next four years, we produced a series of national reports and ran successful conferences for our growing membership. Initially, we attracted only Shadow Ministers to speak, but in 1996 we managed a breakthrough – getting both the Secretary of State for Health and his opposition in the Shadow Cabinet to address our annual conference; one in the morning and the other in the afternoon. I simply phoned their diary secretaries one day to say the other one was coming, and we did not want to deprive their boss the opportunity to give his side of the political debate. Of course, they did not check our claim by phoning each other, and both took the bait. What the two said was of little significance because that we could guess; one broadly supportive and the other politely dismissive. But the point of our invitation was credibility. With them came the press, and with the media came much-needed publicity for our cause.

By 1997, there were at least 135 GP commissioning groups within the UK, involving over 11 000 GPs and 22 million patients, or about a third of the population. Meanwhile, fundholding had just nudged over 50%, albeit using increasingly dilute versions of the scheme to attract increasingly reluctant practices. That May, Labour won the election and Frank Dobson replaced Stephen Dorrell as Secretary of State for Health. There was much discussion about what the new government would do about fundholding and the internal market. It scheduled a White Paper for the end of the year in which policy would be laid out. Remarkably, for the first time, we were invited to contribute formally to a government's thinking, and even received DoH funding to produce a report. Suddenly, our light was on in the corridors of power. It was a strange feeling.

A few weeks later, we published *Restoring the Vision: Making Health the Incentive*.[171] The report sought to refocus attention on the principles of the NHS, for collaboration between all those involved in healthcare, and for incentives for change to be based on professional values rather than financial levers. On the first page, we set out our vision:

> *To develop a comprehensive NHS that is fair to those who use it and those who work within it, efficient and effective in its use of resources, sensitive to the needs of individuals and communities, and openly accountable for its actions.*

It proposed that there should be inclusive, multiprofessional LCGs working within a concept we termed "cooperative commissioning".

Restoring the Vision received praise from many quarters, including the new government. Certainly, many of its themes could be found in the White Paper titled *The New NHS: Modern, Dependable*,[172] which was published three months later. Little known was that a few months before the election, the NACGP executive had met Stephen Dorrell, Secretary of State for Health, and that he had agreed to fund 20 pilots of locality commissioning, allocating £6 million for the exercise. It was a huge moral victory, the first time our approach had ever been nationally recognised, supported, and centrally financed, and it was the Conservative Party that did so.

Not to be outdone, the new government doubled up on Stephen Dorrell's decision, launching 40 locality commissioning pilots across the country in April 1998. These became the prototypes for the PCGs

---

[171] National Association of Commissioning GPs (1997). *Restoring the Vision: Making Health the Incentive*. Nottingham, NACGP.
[172] Department of Health (1997). *The New NHS: Modern, Dependable*. London, Stationery Office.

introduced a year later. But by then, its sole job done, the NACGP had ceased to exist.

We closed our virtual doors on Saturday, 16 May 1998. The NACGP had been a crusade concerning dramatic changes in the NHS. We saw the reforms as useful in many ways, but problematic in others. We had come up with an alternative strategy that had a significant influence on the new Labour government's White Paper. More remarkably, we had also persuaded the previously hostile Conservative government to fund pilot studies of our methods. We acted as a focal point for like-minded people at a time of intense central pressure to adopt a system most GPs disliked and believed to be against the long-term interests of patients and the NHS. As we saw it, we kept a lamp burning within the NHS for equity and cooperation, in contrast to inequity and competition. Fortunately, it was still alight when there was a change of government.

***

The achievements of the fundholding scheme were significant, though not always in the way ministers had intended. Especially in the first and second waves, there were those who made very good use of the opportunities to benefit the care of their patients. Inevitably, proponents of the scheme held up these exceptions as being typical and journalists, in particular, swallowed the press releases without critical inspection. Without fundholding, health authorities would have been the sole purchasers of secondary care, and in the main it seems likely that their managers would have dominated the process, at best giving GPs a notional role as an advisory committee. Many former fundholders still feel that to be a good description of GP commissioning groups, and in some places, unfortunately, they were correct.

The Achilles heel of GP commissioning was its laxity and its lack of accountability. It was the default position for GPs. Even if they agreed to it, there was little to stop a practice ignoring local decisions. And there was little incentive for a health authority to help develop it either. Rather like fundholding, for those at the committed head of the GP commissioning movement it did well, but it had a very long tail. Neither approach had time to mature to allow a realistic, comparative assessment.

It is worth looking at the reasons why such an evaluation was always going to be difficult. Not least, they illustrate how political conviction, by any party, can translate into policies weighed down by loaded dice. And here the dice were both heavy and numerous. As we have seen, the 1990 reforms offered GPs a choice of two ways to become involved in the internal market. But the necessary resources, authority, and support were only made available to one of these. It was the Henry Ford thing; you could choose either option as long as it was the black one. Furthermore, during the first year of the reforms, health authorities were required to continue directly managing the hospitals as before, and were expressly required not to use the internal market! This was to "minimise turbulence" and to allow a "smooth take-off" for fundholders, who meanwhile were receiving additional resources and special training in negotiating skills and management. All this was to help them use the market and compete with health authorities which the government had tied up in a sack. Hospitals themselves were not exempt from external influence to help the political cause. A letter to the *BMJ* in 1994 noted: "Pressure was put on hospitals to increase their throughput from GP fundholders."[173]

Ironically, the purchasing power of DHAs was seen as too big a threat to the whole system. The "small is more powerful" rationalisation of the first fundholding scheme runs counter to normal Tesco-style market principles, and should have sounded alarm bells concerning the government's plans.

---

[173] Sides BA (1994). Fundholding has divided the profession. *BMJ*, 308(6926): 476.

Again, the budgets for health authorities and fundholders were calculated using different formulae. The previous year's spend was used for fundholders, while population size was the determinant for health authority budgets. This crucial difference was presumably unknown to the Secretary of State for Health, Stephen Dorrell, when talking in the House of Commons on 6 February 1996. He said:

> *The resources available to GP fundholders are provided on exactly the same basis as the resources that are available for other forms of patient care.*[174]

That was incorrect.

With such a system, it can be no surprise that there was gaming. For example, some practices prescribed freely in the year preceding their adoption of a fund and used hospital resources generously. Their fund calculation used that unusually high activity, meaning they had a larger fund on starting the following year.[175] Nor should it be surprising that they then made significant "savings" in their first year of fundholding, when their prescribing and referral costs reduced again. Less excusably, these fallacious results were eagerly reported by the press and some academics as demonstrating the merits of fundholding. They were comparing carefully nurtured polished apples with deliberately neglected wild pears, but failing to mention the difference.

All this provides a real-life example of the *Yes Minister*[176] shenanigans that take place when governments press for the uptake of one of various "options" they are offering.

---

[174] *Hansard*: 6 February 1996, vol. 271, cc. 157.

[175] That observation is refuted by some research studies while being supported by others. In the interests of balance, see Harris CM, Scrivener G (1996). Fundholders' prescribing costs: the first five years. *BMJ*, 313(7071): 1531–1534.

[176] The TV series *Yes Minister* follows the ministerial career of Jim Hacker MP and his struggles to formulate and enact legislation while being opposed by the British Civil Service.

***

Nonetheless, fundholding stimulated change in the NHS. It gave the whole service a mighty kick. The kicked jelly not only wobbled; this time, it changed shape. Fundholding was an irritant rather than an end product. It did not take an open mind long to realise that the initial proposals were so flawed as to be non-viable. But without it, locality commissioning might never have evolved to the level it did, perhaps not at all. Hospitals might have sailed on in their customary, imperious manner. Health authorities, as a collective not best-known for Silicon Valley dynamism, may have just soldiered on in their rather bureaucratic manner. And fundholders themselves would not have had the opportunity to develop the idea, notably into multifunds.

Fundholding had a fundamental, strategic benefit that far exceeded the much-trumpeted short-term gains. It catapulted general practice to centre stage of the NHS. It afforded general practice the consideration and resources it required, a necessary change and in my view its greatest achievement. GPs who chose to join the scheme obtained attractive funding for better staff levels, appropriate computer equipment, and direct or indirect help in the development of their premises. Staff, systems, and buildings – the foundation trinity for successful general practice, and the same enhanced resources that followed publication, in 1965, of the BMA's *Charter for the Family Doctor Service*.

Fundholding enabled GPs to be highly innovative, using their fund as a means of developing primary and secondary services for their practice population. The pioneering work of its best exponents offered valuable illustrations of the creative capabilities of GPs. They developed such things as specialist outreach clinics and physiotherapy within their practice premises. Some negotiated faster access for their patients to opinions and operations, though they were egged on to do so by the scheme's advocates, and by hospitals anxious to please them and retain their contracts. Whatever the reason, the result was an act that, by legal contract, contravened the principle of equity within a community.

In various ways, fundholding provided significant benefits for the practices concerned, so why did so many elect to avoid the scheme? Social scientists claim a fundamental difference between the philosophical approaches of fundholders and GP commissioners.[177] If the NHS is about the care of individuals within populations, then fundholders saw their relevant population as the practice list, while GP commissioners extended the "equity within populations" argument out to the locality and health district, though probably not much further than that.

That is an interesting explanation and fits perfectly with discussions I have had with GPs who were fundholders, some of whom readily agreed their focus was on the practice alone. As such, fundholding made perfect sense to them, and yet was anathema to commissioning GPs. It did not make one set of practices good and the other bad; the doctors just held different views on this aspect of the NHS. At best both groups were trying to move forward, to improve things.

Independent studies, such as that of the Audit Commission in 1996, reported that, overall, the fundholding experiment proved expensive for a surprisingly limited benefit.[178] While that may be true in crude economic terms, it does not recognise the collateral lessons I have described, lessons about providing practices with the necessary resources and opportunity to do their job properly; lessons first taught by the document *Our Blueprint for the Future* written by the MPU in 1964, and subsequently *A Charter for the Family Doctor Service*

---

[177] Broadbent J, Jacobs K, Laughlin R (2001). Organisational resistance strategies to unwanted accounting and finance changes: the case of general medical practice in the UK. *AAAJ*, 14(5): 565–586.

[178] Audit Commission (1996). *Fundholding Facts: a Digest of Information About Practices Within the Scheme During the First Five Years*. London, HMSO.

290 · ANDREW WILLIS

produced by the BMA; lessons that could benefit all practices and all patients. It seems fair to conclude that fundholding was successful as a stimulant for change, while being an expensive exercise that was unsustainable in its original form and undesirable in the long term. But the way it highlighted the resources required by general practices, and promoted interagency cooperation concerning commissioning, were things for which we should all be grateful.

***

I mentioned earlier that the original idea of fundholding was fatally flawed, but that it was rescued and developed by the innovations of fundholders themselves. These approaches took various forms.

ECONOMIES OF SCALE

Multifunds were the first significant advance, pooling the funds and endeavour of a group of fundholding practices. They benefited from economies of scale in risk sharing, purchasing leverage, and administration. Covering larger populations, they also reduced inequity of access within a local area. That was still not perfect. While a health authority was by statute responsible for all those within its geographical boundaries, the responsibility of a multifund was limited to the patients registered with its constituent practices. The two were often similar, occasionally very different, and perhaps never the same.[179] In comparison with locality commissioning, they held a partial fund with which they purchased directly; the health authority still bought most of their services. LCGs could only purchase in conjunction with the health authority, but in other ways, the two were

---

[179] As I have already mentioned, in Northampton we considered a district-wide superfund within the OIP project in 1992, to work in cooperation with the DHA, only for the idea to be rejected by the RHA.

very similar. Both were major steps in the evolution of NHS organisation, and both were developed by GPs.

GOING A STRIDE FURTHER

From the fundholding scheme's early days, several leading practices wanted to explore holding an entire budget. In 1994, four were chosen to pilot the idea within the total purchasing pilots (TPPs). By labelling them pilot studies, the NHS circumvented the need for enabling primary legislation, a trick used on various occasions and all too seldom involving study.

The idea was entirely sensible. If the concept of GPs holding a budget is accepted at all, then in economic terms it should be the whole thing and not a mere 20%. If all practices held the entire budget, it would allow the abolition of dual purchasing mechanisms and lead to simplification. Provided population sizes were large enough – a big qualification – it could preserve local equity. It is very much the position of the 2011 policy for CCGs, which also disbanded health authorities.

Within months of the first forays into total purchasing, the NHS executive, flushed with enthusiasm and true to form, expanded the idea without waiting for any objective assessment. It started to recruit a wave of 53 more so-called pilots.

Constitutionally, only a health authority could manage a budget larger than the original 20% figure, and therefore TPPs were made subcommittees of the health authority, which officially managed the budget on behalf of these cuckoos in their nests. In reality, it was total fundholding in all but a legal technicality.

In theory, TPPs combined the best of both worlds: DHA involvement giving strategic direction coupled to the practices' sensitivity to local needs and the individual patient. However, TPPs were still potential loose cannons, capable of threatening the coordination of priorities and purchasing decisions throughout a much larger health district. They still suffered from many of the disadvantages inherent in the original fundholding scheme, such as higher transaction costs, inequity within local populations, and inadequate population size for risk sharing.

That said, along with locality commissioning and multifunds, TPPs helped the development of the next set of organisational contortions within the NHS, the development of PCGs and PCTs. Remarkably, this process was informed by something unusual in NHS progression – a formal, multicentre, academic assessment of the TPP project.[180]

***

It was at this point that the NACGP drew down its blinds. We had used the word commissioning to distinguish ourselves from purchasers, but we had lost the argument to get this distinction accepted universally. Ironically, for most, commissioning now meant purchasing, albeit recognising that needs assessment and outcome review were key components of the process.

Perhaps, at least we could claim some credit for highlighting that there was far more to it than just purchasing. Few used the word commissioning until we coined it, and now it is a commonplace within NHS terminology.[181]

If we were to embrace PCGs and PCTs within our movement, we needed to widen our focus and membership. We needed to include the whole of primary care, nurses and other primary care professionals, social service departments, the voluntary sector, and lay people, in the way that had been promoted, for example, in Northampton's 1994 *A Sense of Place* report.

---

[180] Goodwin N, Mays N, McLeod H, et al. (1998). Evaluation of total purchasing pilots in England and Scotland and implications for primary care groups in England: personal interviews and analysis of routine data. *BMJ*, 317(7153): 256–259.

[181] Typically, the MPU had used it some years earlier, but it was not in common parlance.

For these reasons, the NACGP closed in May 1998, to immediately metamorphose into the NHS Alliance. The Alliance was to be a representative organisation for PCGs and other primary care organisations. Under the diligent helm of its chair, Michael Dixon, and chief executive Mike Sobanja, it developed into a much larger body than its guerrilla group forebear. It had a staff, a professional chief executive, and an executive committee drawn from across the full spectrum of its membership organisations. It reset the movement's purposes and aims, refined them with feedback from around 100 PCGs, and became a significant influence within the NHS.

***

Through all the arguments and counterarguments, the central point of the 1991 reforms remains in place today. Within the NHS, there are now two groups. On the one hand, there are those who provide services, and on the other are those who plan which services are needed, where to get them, how to purchase them, and finally to check that they are delivered to acceptable standards – the four-point plan for doing absolutely anything. However, a substantial pebble remains within this apparently well-oiled market model that divides purchasers from providers, a model born out of policymakers' blinkered obsession with hospitals. GPs are both.

The original fundholding scheme was useful primarily as an irritant. It may have been fundamentally flawed, nonetheless it kick-started beneficial change. It did this largely by prompting GPs, health authorities, and hospitals, supported with greater or lesser enthusiasm by governments, to come up with better models for implementing a market economy.

To conclude this chapter, I recall a 1995 private conversation with a senior civil servant in the DoH. He suggested the methods of delivery would inevitably change and improve; the ferocious debate about fundholding and non-fundholding would cool, with the warring tribes burying their hatchets and coalescing; politicians would come and go as always; but the central strategic core would remain.

Just as in *Yes Minister*, the civil servant was right.

PART SIX

IN THE END

Part Six describes two successful projects within our practice that combined many of the lessons learnt nationally and locally. We had ignored vigorous government preference for our development, because we believed it a threat to the best interests of our patients and the local healthcare community. Inevitably, however, that slowed our progress both in terms of financial support and encouragement. Nonetheless, once we were free to advance again, these projects showed that we managed at least some development.

Finally, the last chapter reflects on the NHS a decade after my retirement.

PUTTING IT ALL INTO PRACTICE

By 1997, our practice had come a long way. We had the infrastructure we wanted regarding people, buildings, and state-of-the art information systems. We were well organised, thanks to excellent managers and staff, and our involvement in major projects both within and outside the practice had given us valuable knowledge and experience. Now, we wanted to put it all together, to ensure we were doing the right thing for the right people in the right way, and to have empirical evidence that we were doing what we intended. In other words, we wanted to use the commissioning cycle of planning, execution, and review with which we were involved within Northampton and nationally, but to do it at a practice level. We still did not want a budget for secondary care; the relevant services remained a tiny element of our work and in any case, we wanted to do pure commissioning in our meaning of the word.

By then, there had been an election, the political climate had changed, and the way forward had been mapped out in the new government's White Paper titled *The New NHS: Modern, Dependable*. It accepted, at least by implication that practices, the core component of the new PCGs, would have to plan, implement, and review services at their own level.

Life had been frustrating for innovative non-fundholders since 1991; we had stagnated, our requests for support and funding having hit a brick wall constructed with political cement. But now, for the first time in seven years, we felt we once more had a chance of central funding for our research and development. We were battle-hardened veterans; we had learnt how to play the game. We presented our proposal as a pilot project.

Those words are relaxing opiates to funding and authorising bodies. Individually, let alone collectively, the words "pilot" and "project" release all manner of restraints applied to less carefully phrased exercises. They huskily whisper "exception" into otherwise cantankerous, bureaucratic ears. "This is an exception; there is no danger of others expecting the same freedom and funding; we can allow this. In fact, it sounds rather a good idea. Why do we not pay for it and claim it as our own?"

THE KING EDWARD ROAD PLANNING AND REVIEW PROJECT

And so it was. Our bid for funding from the NHS executive was successful, though they wanted to expand the project into a broader, national one. They wanted it to involve four other practices, with representatives from fundholding, locality commissioning, total purchasing, and non-fundholding, and to have the whole thing evaluated independently by the University of Manchester.[182] That suited us fine; it was more than we could have hoped for.

Other than being based on a single practice, our project was similar to many GP commissioning groups already at work throughout the country. Inevitably, it was also our perception of the necessary task to be undertaken by a fundholding practice. Its complexity merely emphasised the view that a single practice was, and always had been, too small a population for economically viable commissioning.

We wanted to involve the various skills, disciplines, and experiences within our primary care team and our list of patients, and the expertise and population focus of the District's Department of Public Health, which seconded a senior officer to the project. Also, it

---

[182] National Primary Care Research and Development Centre (1998). *Practice-based Planning and Review: Case Studies of Five GP Practices.* Manchester, National Primary Care Research and Development Centre, University of Manchester.

was supported by its own research worker and our new patient liaison officer, both employed with funds from the project.

We would meld all these subjective opinions with the objective evidence of best practice and set the whole thing within the economic reality of resource constraint. Then, and only then, could the practice decide what services it wanted, what it could best deliver itself, and what should be purchased, directly or indirectly, on its behalf. Objective assessments of the outcomes of our plans would complete the quality assurance cycle.

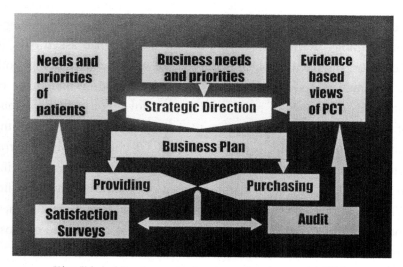

King Edward Road surgery planning and review model 1997.
PCT, primary care trust.

All this was crystallised one memorable Sunday morning in the kitchen, spent with my partner Simon Gregory and a jug of coffee. The result was the above diagram, which to us summarised the commissioning requirements of a practice. Notably, while of course we saw secondary care services as important, they were nonetheless, literally, a secondary matter, and the diagram makes no distinction as to whether it is the practice or some other body that purchases them.

At the beginning of the project, the practice decided on 10 priority areas spread between acute care (for example, access to the practice by telephone, patient education), preventive care (for example, teenage health needs, travel clinics), and chronic disease management (for example, patient compliance with treatment, management of epilepsy). For each, we identified a small task group to gather relevant opinions from within the practice and elsewhere, to blend these with evidence of best practice and public health expertise, and to then come up with viable implementation plans for the practice.

We constructed a computerised resource use profile to help us make sustainable plans and assess outcomes, drawing electronic information reports from the PCT and hospitals concerning our prescribing, and our use of hospital clinics, admissions, pathology, and radiology. Reflecting those questions trainees had asked back in the 1970s, it gave us a much better idea of what we were doing, both as a practice and individually. We were spending hundreds of thousands of pounds of public money, but how? For example, if one of us was referring more patients to a particular department than the others, it could prompt useful discussion. Of course, a high referral rate does not automatically equate to poor practice, much as some like to think it does, any more than it automatically indicates the opposite. What it certainly does is to allow a useful debate among colleagues, and in turn that may prompt behavioural change from some of those involved.

At the same time, we constructed a practice population profile from earlier work with assistance from a colleague who was now at Liverpool University. The profile gave us detailed information about the morbidity and demographics of our patients, for example, mapping where they each lived within the town. Different communities can have very different socio-economic characteristics identified from census and public health data, and these are important determinants of health, and therefore healthcare.

By doing all this, we succeeded in running a full-blown commissioning cycle within our practice, yet without the systems and advantages of being a fundholder. As a team, we had set our priorities, researched each one, and come up with plans for their achievement. Each of those included a clear means of assessing the outcome. All that was a considerable achievement in itself and the results did indeed influence the direction of the practice and alter our clinical behaviour.

It is interesting, in retrospect, to note that none of our 10 priorities involved hospital care. We could have chosen anything, but the main areas we saw for improvement were within the practice, where the majority of our patients' NHS care took place. This echoed a conversation I had with David Colin-Thomé, perhaps the most prominent and successful of the first-wave fundholders. He found the main benefits of the scheme were not in purchasing hospital services, but in having the flexibility and resources to develop the practice itself.

Our project certainly demonstrated how complicated and time-consuming it is to do proper commissioning at a practice level. It added considerable weight to the idea of it being an exercise for groups of practices rather than single ones. In this respect, multifunds, large multipractice TPP schemes, and locality commissioning programmes seemed to have the scale about right.

Having information about what you are doing is, of course, essential for efficient work, but it would be better still if the information allowed comparison with other practices. Single-practice fundholding was a product of a harsh market model, and had no intrinsic provision for such comparison. Larger exercises, such as multifunds and locality commissioning, could do it more easily because practices pooled their resources and effort and, poignantly, because they were working together rather than in competition.

Locality commissioning and our practice-based project offered two valuable lessons. First, it did not require fundholding per se to produce that information at a practice level. Second, it showed that it was too large a task to be undertaken to a high standard in most practices and that it would be better done by a consortium of practices.

The full process of commissioning and strategic planning is not a simple one, even at a locality, PCG/PCT, or CCG level. It had been a long road. Interestingly, the conclusion in Manchester University's report on our project noted:

> *The reforms of the late 1990s influenced the ways in which health services were funded and provided, but made little attempt to integrate the commissioning and provider functions of primary care to create a seamless approach to health care planning.*

The report went on:

> *It was only seven years later that with a change of government and the publication of the 1997 White Paper, strategic planning was placed firmly on the NHS agenda.*

That was a remarkable, independent statement about the so-called reforms of the NHS.

For our part, we had achieved much of what we wanted. We had demonstrated that practice-based planning and review was possible, albeit with considerable difficulty. We had involved all relevant parties in deciding our policies and plans, and we had learnt much about developing appropriate information systems within the practice. But at the end of our two-year project, the NHS had moved on again. PCTs had arrived; they were to be responsible for commissioning on behalf of all the practices in their catchment area. Our task in seclusion was done.

***

PRACTICE MADE PERFECT: RE-ENGINEERING GENERAL PRACTICE

By 2004, the NHS was slowly learning from other service industries and focusing on patients' concerns as well as on what was wrong with them. A tangible benefit of the often-criticised targets and additional money for the NHS at that time was a dramatic reduction in hospital waiting lists. Patients could also now choose the hospital to which they were referred, using the new, electronic Choose and Book system.[183] They could do that if they so wished, but most did not, preferring to take the advice of their GP. That was no surprise; it had been that way in the past.

Meanwhile, general practices were getting in on the act. There was a particular focus on trying to improve access to appointments. As we have seen, there were useful initiatives that made obtaining repeat prescriptions easier; drop-in clinics were opening for commuters away from home, and virtually all practices offered regular review appointments for those with ongoing conditions. The NHS was indeed focusing more on the individual.

In our case, we wanted to take another look at our organisation. There was more and more to be done, partly through increasing demand but more because of the opportunities to offer better prevention and chronic disease management services, and the overbearing volume of administrative work. Indeed, we wanted to take a fresh look at what we were doing and how we were doing it, and then to re-engineer the various processes for improved efficiency and convenience.

Once more, we turned to that trusted, enabling chestnut of proposing a pilot project, dressed up in the sexy terminology of the day: "Practice Made Perfect: Re-engineering General Practice".

---

[183] Choose and Book has been replaced by the NHS e-Referral Service. This was to have started in 2014 but was postponed until 2015 after it failed an assessment by the Government Digital Service.

Intentionally an eye-catching, pretentious title, it was a successful bid that netted an unconditional grant from a helpful and understanding pharmaceutical company.

The idea was simple: there must be more efficient ways to run the practice than were happening already. Our method was that patients, clinicians, and support staff worked together to consider a series of eight case studies, identified the processes involved, and then brainstormed ideas about how to improve things, how to create shortcuts to speed things up, and how to make quality improvements. The following is one example:

> *You are a young mother living alone with your four-year-old son Jack. Jack has woken with a faint rash all over his chest and neck. He is a bit warm, slightly unwell and refuses his breakfast. Jack's father walked out six months ago, and your own family live in another town. You are not sure what to do and need help. You are due to take Jack to the nursery at 8:25 a.m. and then go on to work. You phone the practice at 8:05 a.m., five minutes after it opens.*

At first sight, this looks like an exam question for doctors in training: what is Jack's diagnosis? But that is not the point here. The issue here is not so much the clinical problem as how the mother gets the advice she needs quickly and helpfully. Our task was to think of the problem practically, from the perspectives of patient and practice alike.

We needed to deconstruct the steps involved to see the naked operational issues, and then reconstruct them in as straightforward and efficient a way as possible; to re-engineer the process. When did our phone lines open and how easy would it be for her to get through? Who would, could, or should she speak to when she got through? Was there another way for her to obtain the information she required; a better way? And so on. This was about something other than the traditional model of medicine. It was not the "what" of diagnosis and treatment; it was the "how" of getting the patient the help they required.

We hoped that, at best, the project could bring about startling results by identifying a fundamental, quantum leap simplification of processes. It was not just about creating small improvements. A few percentage points of beneficial changes would hardly justify the project, but a couple of 60% ones could.

Another case concerned the several thousand patients we had on long-term medication. That we wanted to provide them with an excellent repeat medication service was obvious, but how were we going to do that as efficiently and effectively as possible?

> *You are a 45-year-old man who commutes daily to work in London, leaving early and getting home late. You have raised blood pressure that is well controlled with a couple of tablets each day. You take the tablets but are busy, keen to put health issues to one side, and anyway – you are not keen on going to doctors. It irritates you that you have to go through the expensive and inconvenient process of repeat prescriptions every month, even though you only need to get your blood pressure checked twice a year. As it is, you usually have to take a prescription to work and cash it at a London chemist during your lunch break. What you need right now is to organise your next repeat prescription. You phone the practice from work in London to discuss it.*

There is nothing complicated here clinically, but from his point of view, there is plenty. There is a broad range of ways the practice could respond that would affect him.

As mentioned earlier, patient surveys have always shown that what patients most want is an appropriate, empathic, and efficient service. Those are the things our project was all about, and three themes emerged.

THEME 1

The first was to manage the doctors' two conflicting roles. On the one hand, we were directors of the business, attended partnership (board) meetings, and agreed on policy. On the other, we were simply medically qualified members of the practice's team. Here we should be managed like everyone else, by the practice manager, delivering the policies we had agreed as a partnership. The issue here was the natural anarchic, entrepreneurial traits present in many GPs. That is in part what attracted us to the job in the first place, rather than, say, hospital medicine. It is what facilitated the great advances in buildings, systems, staffing, and local health service design described throughout this book. We were self-employed, our own masters.

So, bringing that about would be easier said than done, particularly for the manager, who was our employee. But it was a step towards our acceptance of a corporate approach to managing the practice. The project's consultant adviser, Mike Sobanja,[184] felt it was vital for the future of the practice, indeed for any practice. All the partners could do was to agree our acceptance of the idea, and in the main, we adhered to it.

THEME 2

The second theme concerned how we distributed the work within the team, something traditionally done poorly within general practice. There was a spectrum of tasks to be done, from the purely technical, such as taking a blood pressure reading, through to making decisions, such as analysing multiple new problems presented in a single consultation. Of course, any point on this spectrum needed appropriate

---

[184] Mike Sobanja was Chief Executive of Northampton Health Authority, and then Northamptonshire Health Authority, until 1996. After that, he became Chief Executive Officer of the NHS Alliance, and an independent management consultant.

training, but only the second example required qualification as a doctor. With a doctor costing over four times as much as a healthcare assistant, and roughly three times as much as a practice nurse, no economically astute organisation would employ doctors to do things that others could do equally well at less cost. Five years earlier, I had seen this principle in action during my visit to Kaiser Permanente in California. There, it was unthinkable for an expensive doctor to undertake the administrative and clerical tasks done as routine by NHS GPs. They saw that as throwing away money without reason. Doctors were a valuable, scarce resource, and kept for work that justified their expense.

So, within our project, we decided that, as far as possible, tasks were allocated to appropriately skilled individuals, be they administrative staff, healthcare assistants, nurses, doctors, external agencies, or indeed the patients themselves. So, when patients asked for advice, perhaps from a receptionist or on the telephone, they were transferred to the most appropriate person as quickly as possible.

We agreed on a policy that, under the lead of the senior practice nurse, all preventive care and chronic disease management would be undertaken by practice nurses and healthcare assistants unless the case required specific input from a doctor. This was a significant strategic move, and the numbers were large. For example, in chronic disease management alone, we knew 15% of our patients had an ongoing vascular disease such as heart failure, ischaemic heart disease, peripheral vascular disease, hypertension, stroke, or transient ischaemic attacks, and many had more than one. Again, we knew of 12% who had continuing respiratory conditions, such as asthma or COPD.

We set up specific annual review clinics for chest and vascular conditions, allowing the consideration of related comorbidities and the deployment of appropriate clinical expertise. Although run by our specialist nurses, these two clinics always had a doctor and the practice pharmacist available.

This arrangement was not money grabbing accountancy, but common sense. By ensuring that, within reason, everyone did what only they were trained to do, not only was it more efficient, but it freed doctors and specialist nurses to spend more time with the patients who needed their particular skills. This rule was not an absurd absolute, we did not want petty demarcation disputes, but it was a very useful guideline.

THEME 3

The third theme concerned convenience and efficiency, for patients and the practice alike. It kept cropping up through the project, with references to such things as Web-based communications, telephone consultations, patients being directed quickly and easily to the correct person or service, and expert patient programmes. Here were potentially rich pickings.

We argued that when patients seek medical care, most would prefer not to come to the surgery, if that was possible. As patients, we usually either want information about what to do under a given circumstance (as with the young mother and her son Jack), need to discuss something, or need a practical service, such as a repeat prescription or a blood test (as with the London commuter). In our society's service culture, we want our needs to be met quickly, efficiently, and as effortlessly as possible.

We began to address another simple maxim:

Patients should not come to the surgery, nor we go to them, unless there is no appropriate alternative for providing what they require.

I find helpful the initially alarming idea that you only need to meet a doctor physically if they need to touch you. A discussion over the phone or WWW might prompt a subsequent physical consultation, and we planned consulting space for that, but we knew from experience that more often than not the patient could be managed without it, and to the satisfaction of all concerned.

Of course, that is not an absolute, and there are compelling exceptions. The evaluation of multiple new problems in limited time likely always benefits from clinician and patient being together. Examples in this book include the glanced recognition of the swollen calf of a venous thrombosis; the malignant melanoma spotted during examination of another problem; the grandmother having a heart attack as you glance into the sitting room on the way upstairs to another patient. A phone conversation may focus our attention on what is being said, but conversely we miss visual clues – the body language of distress, the expression on the face of the accompanying relative or friend. Even a camera has a narrower field of vision than the searching human eye. There is no right or wrong way, but there are options, and it is helpful to reconsider the traditional notion that we must always attend the surgery for any form of medical contact.

Such a change would be a significant cultural shift for the practice and for patients, and we only made a start. As operational and societal pressures mount, remote access becomes much more common, just as it has for banks and online shopping.

Equally, we decided to encourage more patients to make use of our electronic systems. These included our website for information, the electronic repeat prescription system, booking appointments online, and recording their arrival using a keypad in reception. For many patients, and not just the younger ones, any or all of these systems proved simple, efficient, and convenient.

Such changes will be driven by patients as much as by practices. The commuter with hypertension would be delighted!

We considered specific areas of our work in the light of those three themes. The first concerned prescribing. As described earlier, we were already involved in a national pilot project concerning the ETP,[185] an opportunity to simplify repeats that was taken up by over 600 of our patients. That alone saved 14 000 contacts a year, but would be substantially extended as more patients took up electronic prescription requests. It would probably suit very nicely the commuter described in the earlier example; when necessary, his tablets could be delivered to his office in London, and at other times to his home. His choice.

Another idea was to extend the duration of each repeat prescription from one month back to perhaps two or three. We had done this since the 1970s but now, to the great displeasure of patients and staff alike, national policy insisted we changed to a monthly duration. Following the project, and swamped with unnecessary repeat prescription requests, we reverted to our old ways and, to everyone's joy doubled the length of most repeat prescriptions. It halved the contacts for those concerned, pleased our patients and staff, and reduced prescription charges for some of them. There was no rise in our overall prescribing costs, and none of us was taken out and shot!

***

So, did "Practice Made Perfect" land a couple of big fish, as we wanted, or just a few tiddlers? Perhaps the greatest benefit arose from the collective exercise of working together and looking at things from the patient's perspective, a focus made easier by having included patients in each of our task groups. It is by such means that cultural changes take place.

But there were definite, tangible benefits. That concerning work distribution was the most profound: the decision to make all chronic disease management and preventive care the responsibility of the

---

[185] Please see the chapter titled "At the Cutting Edge" for a discussion of advanced computer projects.

nursing team, and to inform and support patients in taking control of their own management. At a stroke, the steady crescendo of clinical work within the practice over the previous 30 years was rationalised. We had uncovered swathes of extra work in prevention and in taking back from hospitals the management of ongoing conditions. We the doctors had tried to do it ourselves, but now others would do it. It was a *Back to the Future* moment. Of course, we had started this process already, but now it was formal policy. Now doctors were once more free to spend all their clinical time on the tasks for which only they were trained, while at the same time, the practice provided the full gamut of clinical services.

The project's other big fish involved our efforts to make things more convenient and efficient for patients. These included our tentative steps into distance consulting, use of the WWW for repeat prescribing and booking appointments, and the electronic check-in system on arrival at the surgery. It was only a beginning, though commonplace now, but nonetheless an important step in the right direction.

Unfortunately, the elephant in the room continued to graze undisturbed. The ability to see the doctor you want to see, when you want to see them, remains the Achilles heel of modern-day family medicine. Convenience and efficiency are important, but they should not come at the expense of the empathic, personal approach that patients value so much.

REFLECTIONS IN TINTED GLASS

This book has focused on the period from 1974 to 2006, set within a historical context. How can it be summarised, and what broad lessons could be of benefit in the future, for before we attempt to move forward it may be wise to look back, to see if we have been here before.

There have been benefits that would be unimaginable in the 1960s. Most obvious might be the many new therapies for Parkinson's disease, psychosis, diabetes, asthma, infection, vascular disease, and malignancies; the sophistication of dressings; fluid replacement solutions; and patients having far greater access to the professions allied to medicine, such as physiotherapy and podiatry.

Access to diagnostic investigations has increased, complemented by new specialised techniques such as endoscopy, echocardiography, CT, and MRI scans. The NHS has been transformed by general practice's implementation of preventive medical care and its management of ongoing conditions.

But also important has been a change of approach, from medical paternalism to a more mature, collaborative relationship. It is far from complete, but moving strongly in the right direction. Now, patients help themselves by using modern technologies such as glucometers, peak flow meters, and personal blood pressure machines. They are encouraged to discuss management options and access the maze of information available on the WWW. Public awareness of the effects of lifestyle choices on our health is immeasurably better than in the 1960s, even if some of the advice – such as that concerning dietary sugar intake – is widely ignored.

The scope, organisation, buildings, and staff of general practice have exploded into life. Three national bodies, the RCGP, the BMA, and governments of many colours, contributed to this accelerated evolution though they had different motives.

Politicians, ever the pragmatists, saw opportunities to contain one of their greatest domestic headaches, the insatiable appetite of the NHS. Hospitals have always been by far the largest financial quicksand, with self-employed, relatively autonomous GPs guarding all paths leading to it with variable enthusiasm. What politicians of any party needed was a means of controlling the actions of the independently contracted GPs. Shifting responsibility for most of the budget to these swashbuckling entrepreneurs was a controversial move, but ultimately – despite very real threats to the doctor–patient relationship that have seldom been acknowledged, and once the initial fundamental mistakes were corrected – the market strategy is set to evolve and make better use of resources within the NHS. Clinical generalists are uniquely placed to do that well, provided the NHS recognises and declares that doctors' primary responsibility is to patients, not the Treasury.

The second radical change attributable to politicians is the benefit arising from competition in the broad sense of the word. Goals, targets, objective assessment, and review – call them what you will – humans respond to stimuli. It is a characteristic of life itself: a sunflower rotates its face to follow the sun; an amoeba moves towards a drop of sugar solution. We need a reason to get up in the morning; without that, we do not get up. The most pressing challenge facing NHS policymakers concerns a nearly impossible balance. It is to use all these advances to improve an NHS that remains true to its founding principles while at the same time avoiding the incompatible disadvantages of a crude market.

Although GPs founded their college on altruism, it has risen to give general practice a solid foundation of research and professionalism. The RCGP has also developed the most sophisticated training schemes of any branch of the medical profession, and the most rigorous examination of competence. It has managed to avoid becoming embroiled in politics, which has helped its voice to be heard by policymakers.

Meanwhile, the BMA's equally useful contributions – the Charter, contractual negotiations, espousal of professional standards and ethics – arose from promoting the role and well-being of GPs, the largest group among its members.

So, while their motivation differed, the effects of all three of these major bodies of influence moved general practice forward.

When it comes to discoveries and inventions, one thing above all others has enabled the development of modern general practice. Almost every chapter of this book touches on the benefit of computers and their related technologies. The shift in focus away from the previously dominant hospitals towards primary care, and general practice in particular, reflects the enabling contribution of computers and networks.

But not all has been good. There has been an excessive structural change in the NHS, and much of it has been unhelpful. There have been disadvantages too in a market economy. Cooperation has been tarnished and undermined, yet it was a traditional hallmark of the NHS. An unfettered market can do that, and do it by intent.

Our consumeristic society has become more litigious in general, with unspoken disadvantages for patient care that need weighing against any advantages for individuals. Medical practice so often involves judgement, an opinion based on evaluating incomplete information. Judgement involves risk, and a backdrop of increasing litigation means ever more defensive working. Of course, that has benefits. Clinicians are more attentive to detail, and they are more certain and precise. But it also has disadvantages: excessive caution can lead to delay; unnecessary investigations convey costs and inconvenience for patients and the service; and ultimately unnecessary treatments may bring iatrogenic sequelae.

Another change that has strengths and weaknesses is the loss of the GP 24-hour commitment. These extend beyond the social niceties for patients and doctors. Fatigue dulls performance – an example from another field is research showing that driver fatigue caused 20% of UK road accidents. Doctors doing intellectually challenging work while stressed and working very long shifts of duty are at increased risk of making mistakes. It is often during unsocial hours that we patients need urgent help; we used to call a doctor from their bed to provide that emergency medical care. That was dangerous.

I remember getting up in the 1980s to drive, bleary-eyed, round Northampton's ring road at 3:00 a.m., only to bounce off the kerb of a roundabout. It could have been nasty, but no harm accrued other than to my rim and tracking. It was not that I had fallen asleep at the wheel; I had not woken up. At least, it roused me in time to give the patient due attention a few minutes later. (The whole incident was absurd. I was driving across town simply to take a couple of paracetamol tablets to a patient who had severe toothache, and apparently had no painkillers in the house. Their phone call had lobbed me a ticking bomb, as referred to in an earlier chapter. I had no option but to act. Times have changed since then.) For a while following that incident, I put a wet facecloth by my bed when I was on duty, an act akin to the proverbial wet fish but cheaper and less inclined to smell. Plan, resource, do, review.

As with so many things, the cessation of the 24-hour contract was a balance. It was right that the soft factors of empathy and familiarity were trumped by the hard reality of safety for patients and acceptable working conditions for their doctors, no matter how much we value the former.

It was also to the convenience of those watchful, pragmatic politicians. They must have shed crocodile tears as the independent contractor GPs negotiated away their medical monopoly. It let competition from other providers into the previously impenetrable fortress of general practice. Two historical foundations of general practice had gone: the GP monopoly that meant they were largely untouchable because no one else would take on the total commitment, and the open-ended funding of services for their patients. The erosion of that started in the 1970s, but it was only with practice-level budgets that constraint began to bite.

Standardisation is another issue that has good and bad characteristics. Practices and clinical behaviour have both converged in their separate if overlapping evolutions, as have modern cars or franchised food outlets. There is less freedom to innovate. A loss of individuality is the price we pay for consistency. In medicine, overall, it is a price worth paying. If the NHS is to pursue equity and quality for all, it has no choice but to draw up the worse providers to the levels of the more successful ones. Again, this emphasises the difference between a pure competitive market and an organisation with a broader mandate, one that is truly socially aware. The NHS, with its focus on quality and equity for patients, is too subtle an organism for a free market. For sure, the NHS has a responsibility to produce winners, but at the same time it must also ensure there are no losers. If taken as an absolute, such a zero-sum game makes impossible demands of policymakers within the principled boundaries of the NHS, but it is a worthy guiding principle.

It is important to recognise the different, if overlapping, agendas of patients, professions, and politicians. It is not that one group is right and another wrong, but we should be consistent. It is wrong to talk about the vested interests of the professions and BMA – a favoured populist slur from politicians and journalists – if politicians fail to mention at the same time their own vested interests in economic consideration, let alone ideology, or if journalists fail to acknowledge the requirements for brevity and speed in their task. It is also unfortunate, if far more understandable, when a patient or their advocate fails to recognise that their personal perspective must fit a broader view. These are all different agendas, but all valid. The trick is for all parties to be sensitive to each other's wants and needs, to agree what they are trying to do collectively in any particular circumstance, and then to set about doing it.

There is another important spectrum of opinion, the self–society axis. At one end are those with a sole interest in the self, and at the other those with a total commitment to society. Most of us are somewhere in between. An appreciation of this spectrum helps us understand the views of different people. For example, it is remarkably apt regarding political views on healthcare in the USA.

Another clear lesson is that if generalists have the tools and opportunity to expand their work, they will grasp them, innovate, and deliver beneficial change. At the same time, it is important to recognise yet another range, stretching from the highly innovative at one end to the highly tardy at the other. Again, most inhabit the centre of the bell-shaped curve, watching developments and using the best of the innovations to enhance their work. But that variation is unacceptable to those with an interest in correcting health inequalities. They will reach for rules of standardisation, the route governments have taken since the turn of the century. We have already considered the unintended, perverse consequence of tightening the tap on creativity and innovation.

Much as some do not like a market economy in healthcare, they have failed to come up with solid, alternative proposals. Increasing demand for an unrestricted range of services, free at the point of use, cannot be paid for with a finite budget that rises more slowly than the escalation in costs. That equation is unstable, untenable. Whether they like it or not, this is a conundrum that politicians must address themselves. They cannot shift the blame of rationing to clinicians who have their own, different responsibilities. But it follows that it is beholden on those without that prodigious national responsibility to give policymakers space and time to enact their plans, provided those are transparent and open to critical consideration.

***

All that happened over the course of a single career. It happened for all of us who qualified in the late 1960s and early 1970s. The following 30–40 years saw a seismic shift, the creation of something vastly different to anything that had gone before. These were the early years of modern general practice within the NHS.

***

After all those general reflections about the service at large, I will finish from an individual's perspective. What were the two key moments for me, personally, during the span of my career? Both would be clinical, despite my love for toys and for over three decades swimming in the invigorating sea of technical change.

The first was that final consultation, the one on the morning I retired. I knew the patient well, and we were both well aware she was only a few hours from the end of her life. It was the final consultation, literally, for both of us. It was a success, and it did not matter to either of us that no textbook medicine was involved at all. There is more to medical practice than that.

And the second? It was an evening in hospital; a quietly spoken Australian surgeon sat on the side of my bed. I was 33 with a young family and a large mortgage, and concerned I might die. Just the two of us, alone, we talked about my brain tumour and what he was going to do about it. Somehow, he gained my immediate and complete trust. Then and there, I learnt the truth of a quotation I had long known and liked:

The essential unit of medical practice is the occasion when, in the intimacy of the consulting room or sick room, a person who is ill, or believes himself to be ill, seeks the advice of a doctor whom he trusts. This is the consultation, and all else in the practice of medicine derives from it.[186]

That may well have been true in 1960. Certainly, it was true in the days of William Barr and Robert Bradley Roe, and it was true at the start of this book. But I hope I have shown that now it is not so simple. The delivery of healthcare is no longer just about the individual. I prefer to meld Sir James Spence's elegant words with the subtly differing concept I learnt from Kaiser Permanente in California, that of "providing comprehensive healthcare to populations, one patient at a time."

If we can combine those two descriptions with economic efficiency, adequate funding, high standards, and the enduring principles of the NHS applied to the whole population, then we will indeed have a health service of which we can all be proud.

***

My hope is that this book accurately reflects the times and events of the 32 years spanning my career. Even with the best of intentions, it is all too easy to be ambiguous or to mislead. So, my final anecdote displays that fact, and involves the mind-bender par excellence, the bringer of gaiety and sorrow, and the most socially acceptable of all drugs of addiction: alcohol.

When I was a junior hospital doctor in Salisbury, we would occasionally prescribe a nightcap for older patients: a sherry for her and a Guinness for him, all on the NHS. After all, they were far better than the alternative barbiturate sedatives.

---

[186] Spence Sir James Calvert (1960). *The Purpose and Practice of Medicine.* Oxford, OUP, pp. 273–274.

How times have changed![187]

But I never lost the idea. Towards the end of my career, I was visiting a sweet old lady in one of the "poet streets" of Northampton. I called them that; there were Chaucer, Byron, and Shelley at least. The patient had trouble getting off to sleep and did not like tablets. I suggested she got a bottle of sherry and tried that before bed.

A month later I returned, and among other things enquired if she had found any benefit from the sherry.

"Yes I did, doctor, thank you. But I must confess – I could not manage the whole bottle before I fell asleep."

---

[187] Again in the early 1970s, our paediatricians in Northampton occasionally prescribed asthmatic children a two-week holiday in the mountains of Switzerland for "fresh air" and to "get away from it all". What it was they were getting away from was never overtly stated, and I never knew who funded the trips, or where the children stayed.

LIST OF ABBREVIATIONS

BASIC	Beginner's All-purpose Symbolic Instruction Code
BMA	British Medical Association
CCG	clinical commissioning group
CEO	chief executive officer
CGP	College of General Practitioners
DGH	district general hospital
DHA	district health authority
DoH	Department of Health
DTI	Department of Trade and Industry
ETP	Electronic Transfer of Prescriptions
FHSA	family health service authority
FPC	family practitioner committee
GMSC	General Medical Services Committee
GP	general practitioner
HCHS	hospital and community health services
ICU	intensive care unit
LCG	locality commissioning group
MPU	Medical Practitioners' Union
NACGP	National Association of Commissioning GPs
NHS	National Health Service (UK)
NSF	National Service Framework
OIP	Options in Purchasing [project]
OSI	Open Systems Interconnection
PCG	primary care group
PCT	primary care trust
PHCT	primary health care team
PPA	Prescription Pricing Authority
PSG	patient support group
QOF	Quality and Outcomes Framework
RCGP	Royal College of General Practitioners

RCP	Royal College of Physicians
RHA	regional health authority
RHB	regional hospital board
RPI	retail price index
SLG	specialty liaison group
TPP	total purchasing pilot
WWW	World Wide Web

INDEX

(Page numbers in italics denote figures. Text in italics denotes publication titles. Footnotes are shown in the format "320 n187", that is, page number 320, footnote 187.)

ABOUT THE AUTHOR

Throughout his 32-year career, Andrew Willis was a partner in the same Northampton practice. At different times, he also worked as a hospital clinical assistant in rheumatology, a visiting GP to an adolescent psychiatric unit, for Northampton Health Authority as its liaison GP, for Northamptonshire FHSA as a consultant in general practice, and – conveniently, while his children were young – as industrial doctor for the Mettoy toy factory.

Following government reforms of the NHS in 1989, he was involved in planning local and national services, becoming chair of the NACGP in 1994, and then the first president of the NHS Alliance.

His enthusiasm for developing general practice spanned its buildings, information systems, organisation, and personnel.

In 1991, he was awarded a Master in Social Science degree for his work on the information needs of general practices, and the following year he achieved Fellowship by Assessment of the RCGP.

In retirement, much of his spare time is still consumed by designing and making things, whether in photography, gardening, or woodwork. His wife Eunice is also a retired GP; they moved to Chester in 2014. They have three children and seven grandchildren.

Lightning Source UK Ltd.
Milton Keynes UK
UKOW05f0140240217
295212UK00008B/102/P